AF903411

SEXUAL DYSFUNCTIONS – SPECIAL ISSUES

Edited by **Azita Goshtasebi**

Sexual Dysfunctions – Special Issues
Edited by Azita Goshtasebi

Published by InTech

Janeza Trdine 9, 51000 Rijeka, Croatia

Copyright © 2011 InTech

All chapters are distributed under the Creative Commons Attribution 3.0 license, which allows users to download, copy and build upon published articles even for commercial purposes, as long as the author and publisher are properly credited, which ensures maximum dissemination and a wider impact of our publications. After this work has been published by InTech, authors have the right to republish it, in whole or part, in any publication of which they are the author, and to make other personal use of the work. Any republication, referencing or personal use of the work must explicitly identify the original source.

As for readers, this license allows users to download, copy and build upon published chapters even for commercial purposes, as long as the author and publisher are properly credited, which ensures maximum dissemination and a wider impact of our publications.

Notice

Statements and opinions expressed in the chapters are these of the individual contributors and not necessarily those of the editors or publisher. No responsibility is accepted for the accuracy of information contained in the published chapters. The publisher assumes no responsibility for any damage or injury to persons or property arising out of the use of any materials, instructions, methods or ideas contained in the book.

Publishing Process Manager Dejan Grgur

Technical Editor Teodora Smiljanic

Cover Designer InTech Design Team

Additional hard copies can be obtained from orders@intechopen.com

Sexual Dysfunctions – Special Issues, Azita Goshtasebi
p. cm.
ISBN 978-953-307-859-5

We are IntechOpen,
the world's leading publisher of
Open Access books
Built by scientists, for scientists

4,000+
Open access books available

116,000+
International authors and editors

120M+
Downloads

151
Countries delivered to

Our authors are among the
Top 1%
most cited scientists

12.2%
Contributors from top 500 universities

WEB OF SCIENCE™

Selection of our books indexed in the Book Citation Index
in Web of Science™ Core Collection (BKCI)

Interested in publishing with us?
Contact book.department@intechopen.com

Numbers displayed above are based on latest data collected.
For more information visit www.intechopen.com

For EU product safety concerns:
IN TECH d.o.o., Prolaz Marije Krucifikse Kozulić 3, 51000 Rijeka, Croatia,
info@intechopen.com or visit our website at intechopen.com.

Meet the editor

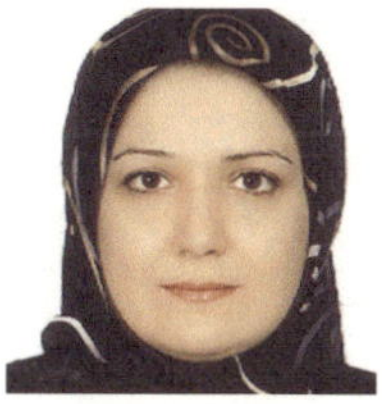

Dr. Azita Goshtasebi, MD, PhD is a Mother and Child Health Specialist at the Iranian Institute for Health Sciences Research, ACECR in Tehran, Iran. As a pioneer in the field, she has focused her research interest on sexual and reproductive health, especially female sexual dysfunctions. She is a passionate advocate for incorporating sexual health into medical curricula. Having published and reviewed several papers, book chapters and books, Dr. Goshtasebi has become widely recognized for her education and practice expertise in sexual and reproductive health.

Contents

Preface

Scientists and public health professionals are beginning to acknowledge sexual health and its role in reproductive and mental health of people. Sexual dysfunctions are common and have psychological and social consequences. As suggested by the title, the book "Sexual Dysfunctions - Special Issues" represents a painstaking analysis of some of the issues in the field that are worth mentioning.

The target audiences for the book are those health care providers who are interested in sexual and reproductive health, clinicians who treat chronic diseases that affect sexuality to some extent, and researchers who would like to study epidemiology, pathophysiology and treatment of sexual dysfunctions.

The main goal of this book is to provide a new perspective on sexual dysfunctions through contribution of experts from different disciplines.

The literature on sexual dysfunctions is relatively limited worldwide. Thus, the first section presents a systematic review of the prevalence of sexual dysfunctions in men and women along with the associated subjects in this area.

Many patients and medical professionals assume that sexual functions are not of concern in chronic diseases. For example, cancer survivors were so busy with the treatment and its side effects that they never thought about their sexual life. However, the truth is that sexuality is a major concern even in disabled patients, and should be integrated in the management plan of patients. Sexual function and dysfunction in some medical conditions is discussed in Section two.

Sexual dysfunctions were considered to be merely a psychological matter for many years. Experimental studies using animal models have made a remarkable contribution to changing this perception and have had a significant part in studying physiology and treatment of sexual dysfunctions. The last section provides some examples of these studies, which might be of interest to investigators of sexual function and dysfunction.

There are many related topics that are not included in this edition, which will surely be addressed in the revisions. It is my hope that the readers will find this book to be valuable and practical in education, research and treatment of sexual dysfunctions.

Azita Goshtasebi
Department of Family Health, Mother and Child Health Research Center,
Iranian Institute for Health Sciences Research, ACECR
Tehran,
Iran

Part 1

Epidemiology of Sexual Dysfunctions

1

Prevalence of Sexual Dysfunctions: A Systemic Approach

Azita Goshtasebi[1], Samira Behboudi Gandevani[2], and Abbas Rahimi Foroushani[3]
[1]*Department of Family Health, Mother and Child Health Research Center, Iranian Institute for Health Sciences Research, ACECR, Tehran,*
[2]*Midwifery Department, Faculty of Medicine, Tarbiat Modares University, Tehran,*
[3]*Department of Epidemiology and Biostatistics, Faculty of Public Health, Tehran, University of Medical Sciences, Tehran,*
Iran

1. Introduction

This chapter is intended to provide an evidence-based overview of the worldwide epidemiology of sexual dysfunction since the 1990s in general populations of different countries, allowing for the generalization of findings at the given population level. The descriptive and analytic literature on sexual function was identified through searching conventional databases, literature surveys and references. This chapter is organized as follows: we first review epidemiological concepts focusing on the issue of determining prevalence; then, we review the female and male sexual dysfunctions prevalence.

Since only recently sexual function and sexual problems have been openly discussed in most societies and cultures (Tiefer, 2001), few epidemiologic data exist until the middle of the twentieth century. The large population-based study of normative data on female sexuality was published by Kinsey and coworkers in 1953. Recent studies, however, have presented a more accurate picture of sexual dysfunction prevalence.

2. The epidemiology of sexual dysfunction

Epidemiology is a scientific study of the distribution and determinants of diseases in populations. Epidemiological data are the basis for assessing the overall impact of a condition on a given society (Prins et al., 2002). These data are needed for public health systems in order to recognize the impact of the studied condition in the population and organize screening, diagnostic and treatment strategies .One of the basic epidemiological measures of outcome occurrence is *prevalence* which is defined as the proportion of a population exhibiting a health condition during a specific time interval (Simons et al. 2001). Moreover, prevalence is characterized by the proportion of a given population which has the condition at a given time. While prevalence can refer to any time period, researchers typically distinguish among point, period and lifetime prevalence. An important conceptual issue is to define sexual dysfunction which is used when it is clinically diagnosed. Another issue is to select the study sample. Community-based samples are the most appropriate ones which define the potential number of patients sustaining the disorder/condition who might benefit from treatment. The study sample must be a representative of the studied population in terms of social, cultural and health status. And, the last one is to select the tools used for screening.

In this chapter, the criterion was the prevalence estimate for general populations, which included a representative sample of community with overall methodological quality. The internal validity of the study was assessed by data collection procedures, measurement instruments, defining health conditions and informative content of reported prevalence. External validity was assessed by the generalizability of the study and source of population, sampling, eligibility of criteria and response rate (Tsai et al, 2011).

The second important issue is that sexual dysfunction may be best conceptualized as the global inhibition of sexual response due to interpersonal factors (Hartmann et al, 2002) because many cases of sexual dysfunction can be regarded as the adaption to sexual relationship problems. In other words, sexual dysfunction must be seen in a multi-faceted socio-psycho-biologic context. Therefore, there are different scales for defining and classifying sexual dysfunction including the American Psychiatric Association's Diagnosis and Statistical Manual for Mental Disorder, 4th text revision (DSM-III or IV-TR), the World Health Organization's International Classification of Diagnosis (ICD-10), Profile of Female Sexual Function(PFSF), Female Sexual Function Index (FSFI), Golombok Rust Inventory of Sexual Satisfaction (GRISS), International Index of Erectile Function (IIEF), Sexual Function Questionnaire (SFQ) and other researcher-made validated questionnaires . Clearly, the type of applied definition affects the prevalence estimate of sexual problems. Although the database in both groups is rapidly growing, in this chapter, we tried to include all the recent studies of the field.

We focused on epidemiologic studies on sexual problems, sexual disorders or sexual distress which have estimated prevalence of one or more sexual problems for general populations in the world. Thus, we excluded studies with a small sample size and studies in special populations like specific health conditions.

In this review, we searched MEDLINE, SCIENCEDIRECT, PUBMED, GOOGLE SCHOLAR, JSTORE and JSTORE PROQUEST using the following key words: epidemiology, prevalence plus sexual dysfunction, sexual function disturbance, sexual disorder, dyspareunia, vaginismus, anorgasmia, lack of lubrication, sexual arousal, sexual desire, hypoactive sexual desire disorder, sexual aversion disorder, orgasmic disorder, erectile dysfunction, early ejaculation and premature ejaculation.

3. Prevalence of female sexual dysfunction

Despite increasing scientist interest in female sexual difficulty and dysfunction, the true prevalence of female sexual dysfunctions (FSD) in the general population remains a contentious issue. One reason is the great deal of variation in the published prevalence estimates of female sexual difficulties/ dysfunctions. This variation may be due, in part, to real differences among populations, and the way FSD is measured (Lindau et al,. 2007). Lack of standardization of outcome measures is an important issue in the FSD literature which has been raised by previous authors. Also, different time frames have influenced the prevalence rate. If the period of study increases, prevalence increases, too (Mercer et al,. 2003).

The prevalence of female sexual dysfunctions, as reported in reasonably valid descriptive investigations, are showed in Tables 1-4. There are currently four international data sets with some information about women's sexual problem; five studies in Africa, eleven studies in Asia, eleven studies in Europe and eleven studies in America.

3.1 Sexual interest/desire dysorders

Table 1 show that the low level of sexual desire prevails in 11.2%-66.4% of subjects in different age strata. This indicates that sexual arousal dysfunction with this large variation is a worldwide problem at different ages. In several countries, there is a clear decline in sexual interest at advanced ages.

3.2 Arousal/lubrication dysorders

There are genital and psychological aspects for arousal disorders. But, they are not explicitly separated. Insufficient lubrication generally appears in almost 49% of women. Also, it seems that this problem is more common in two ends of reproductive ages.

3.3 Orgasm dysorders

The prevalence of orgasmic dysfunction varies considerably within and between different geographic areas and some researchers believe that this problem may or may not be age-dependent. The highest report belongs to India in which more than 86% of women report this problem. Also, this problem is very common among African women.

3.4 Dyspareunia

The manifest of genital pain during intercourse has been also reported by a large number of women all over the world. Overall, high prevalence of about 64% has been found in Asia and Africa.

Vaginismus is another painful condition during intercourse with high prevalence in Asia. But, it appears that there is clear lack of investigation of this problem in the world.

4. Prevalence of male sexual dysfunction

Male sexual dysfunction includes erectile dysfunction (ED), ejaculation disorders, orgasmic dysfunctions and disorders of sexual interest/desire. Epidemiologic studies have supported the high prevalence of male sexual dysfunction worldwide; however, the data are limited. Many of the epidemiologic studies are old and related to poor methodology. In this chapter, we reviewed 29 multiethnic studies about these problems. Tables 1-4 show validated studies on the prevalence of male sexual dysfunction.

4.1 Erectile dysfunction (ED)

Erectile dysfunction (ED) is defined as the consistent or recurrent inability of a man to attain and/or maintain penile erection sufficiently for a sexual activity. A 3-month minimum duration is accepted for the establishment of the diagnosis. Several studies have provided data on the prevalence of ED. The prevalence of ED on a worldwide basis has a great deal of variation around 9%-69%. And, there is a clear increase of this disorder at older ages. In all studies, ED has a rather high rate from 20% to 40% for the ages 60 to 69 years old, some increasing after the age of 65 years old.

4.2 Ejaculation disorders

Ejaculation disorders include early ejaculation, delayed ejaculation and anejaculation. The term early ejaculation is used to replace premature ejaculation, a term considered relatively inaccurate and pejorative. Early ejaculation is the ejaculation that occurs sooner than desired, either before or shortly after penetration, over which the sufferer has minimal or no control. Like all or most other dysfunctions, this is primarily a self-reported diagnosis. Delayed ejaculation is the undue delay in reaching a climax during sexual activity. Anejaculation is the absence of ejaculation during orgasm (Althof et al, 2006).

The major problem in assessing the prevalence of early ejaculation is lack of an accurate (validated) definition. It can be defined by time of ejaculation, in the context of the sufferer's or partner's satisfaction, the number of penile thrusts after intromission or even in the context of the amount of sexual stimulation. Similarly, there is lack of definition for the delayed ejaculation. The highest prevalence rate of 31% (men aged 18-59 years old) was given by the NHSLS study in the United States (Laumann et al., 1999). In the sub-groups aged 18 to 29, 30 to 39, 40 to 49 and 50 to 59 years old, the prevalence was 30%, 32%, 28% and 55%, respectively. These high prevalence rates may be a result of the dichotomous scale (yes/no) in a single question asking whether the ejaculation occurred too early or not.

4.3 Orgasmic dysfunction

Orgasmic dysfunction is the inability in achieving orgasm, markedly diminished intensity of orgasmic sensations or marked delay of orgasm during conscious sexual activity. There is a self-report of high sexual arousal/excitement in this disorder. Prevalence data on orgasmic dysfunction are scarce and report 5%-33% of all men in the world. One simple reason explaining the difficulty of assessing the prevalence of orgasmic dysfunction is that some men may be unable to distinguish between ejaculation and orgasm.

4.4 Sexual interest/desire dysfunctions

Sexual interest/desire dysfunctions are diminished or no feelings of sexual interest or desire, no sexual thoughts or fantasies and lack of responsive desire. This problem has been neglected in epidemiologic studies to some extent; but it is quite commonly seen in clinical practices. The prevalence rate of sexual interest disorders is 11%-28% around the world. The highest prevalence rate of sexual interest disorders was reported in a study conducted in Asia in men aged 40 to 80 years old. It seems that there is not any pronounced age effect on this problem. However, more research would shed more light on this issue.

	Problem or question	Sample size	Scale	Cohort age (year)	Prevalence (%)
Female					
Amidu et al, 2011		301	GRISS	18-58	
	Overall sexual problems				72.8
	Anorgasmia				72.4
	Sexual infrequency				71.4
	Dissatisfaction				77.7
	Vaginismus				68.1
	Avoidance of sexual intercourse				62.5

Laumann et al, 2005		967	Ad hoc questionnaire	40-80	
	Lack of sexual interest				43.4
	Inability to reach orgasm				23
	Orgasm too quickly				10
	Pain during sex				21
	Lubrication difficulties				23
Elnashar et al, 2007		936	Ad hoc questionnaire	16-49	
	Dyspareunia				31.5
	Decreased sexual desire				49.6
	Difficult arousal				36
	Anorgasmia				16.9
Kadri et al, 2002		728	DSM-IV	20-80	
	Overall sexual dysfunction				26.6
	Hypoactive sexual desire				18.3
	disorder				15
	Sexual aversion disorder				12
	Orgasmic disorder				8.3
	Sexual arousal disorder				7.5
	Dyspareunia				6.2
	Vaginismus				
Hassanin et al, 2010		601	Ad hoc questionnaire	18-60	
	Overall sexual dysfunction				76.9
	Low sexual desire				66.4
	Dyspareunia				64
	Sexual dissatisfaction				54
	Lack of lubrication				53
	Low sexual arousal				57
	Orgasmic disorder				61
Male					
Seyam et al, 2003		805	Ad hoc questionnaire		
	Erectile dysfunction			20+	10.3
				50-59	26
				60-69	49
				70-79	52
Amidu et al, 2011		255	GRISS	19+	
	Overall sexual dysfunction				66
	Premature ejaculation				64.7
	Impotency				59.6
	No sensuality				59.2
	Avoidance				49

GRISS: Golombok Rust Inventory of Sexual Satisfaction
DSM-IV: Diagnosis and Statistical Manual for Mental Disorder, 4th

Table 1. Characteristics of African studies of sexual dysfunction

	Problem or question	Sample size	Scale	Cohort age (year)	Prevalence (%)
Female					
Shifren et al, 2008		31581	CSFQ-14	18+	
	Low desire				37.7

	Low arousal Low orgasm Any (desire, arousal or orgasm)				25.3 21.1 43.1
Lindau et al, 2007	Low desire Difficulty with vaginal lubrication Inability to climax	1550	Ad hoc questionnaire	57-85	43 39 34
Laumann et al, 2005	Lack of sexual interest Inability to reach orgasm Orgasm too quickly Pain during sex Pain during sex	1845	Ad hoc questionnaire	40-80	32.9 25.2 10.5 14 27.1
Bancroft et al, 2002	Lubrication problems Pain disorders No orgasm	987	DSM-IV	20-65	31 3 9
Addis et al, 2006	Overall sexual dysfunction	2109	Ad hoc questionnaire	40-69	24
Laumann et al, 2008	Lacked interest in sex	1550	Ad hoc questionnaire	57-64 65-74 75-85	45.4 37.6 49.3
	Unable to achieve orgasm			57-64 65-74 75-85	35 33.4 38.2
	Experienced pain during sex			57-64 65-74 75-85	18.2 18.9 11.8
Abdo et al, 2004	Lack of sexual desire Pain during sexual intercourse Orgasmic dysfunction	1219	Ad hoc questionnaire	18+	26.7 23.1 21
Laumann et al, 1999	Overall sexual dysfunction	1749	DSM-IV	18-59	43
	Lacked Interest in Sex			18-29 30-39 40-49 50-59	32 32 30 27
	Unable to Achieve Orgasm			18-29 30-39 40-49 50-59	26 28 22 23
	Experienced Pain During Sex			18-29 30-39 40-49 50-59	21 15 13 8
	Difficulty in Lubricating			18-29 30-39 40-49 50-59	19 18 21 27

West et al, 2008	Low Sexual Desire Hypoactive Sexual Desire Disorder	2207	PFSF	30-70	36.2 8.3
Junior et al, 2005	Lubrication difficulties Lack of sexual interest	728	Ad hoc questionnaire	40-80	23.4 22.7
Male					
Lindau et al, 2007	Erectile difficulties	1455	Ad hoc questionnaire	57-85	37
Laumann et al, 2005	Lack of sexual interest Inability to reach orgasm Early ejaculation Pain during sex Erectile difficulties	2205	Ad hoc questionnaire	40-80	17.6 14.5 27.4 3.6 20.6
Laumann et al, 2008	Lacked interest in sex	1550	Ad hoc questionnaire	57-64 65-74 75-85	27.8 28.7 24.4
	Unable to achieve orgasm			57-64 65-74 75-85	16.1 22.9 33
	Experienced pain during sex			57-64 65-74 75-85	3 3.2 1
Derby et al, 2000	Erectile dysfunction	505	IIEF BMSFI	50-70	18 8
Ansong et al, 2000	Erectile dysfunction	5198	Ad hoc questionnaire	50-76 50-54 55-59 60-64 65-69 70-76	46.3 26 34.9 46.9 57.8 69.4
Moreira et al, 2001	Erectile dysfunction	1286	Ad hoc questionnaire	18+	46.2
Saigal et al, 2006	Erectile dysfunction	3566	Ad hoc questionnaire	20+ 20-29 30-39 40-49 50-59 60-69 70-74 ≥75	12.3 4.7 3.4 7 19.9 27 38 30
Johannes et al, 2000	Erectile dysfunction	1156	Ad hoc questionnaire	40-69 40-49 50-59 60-69	25.9 12.4 29.8 46.4

Laumann et al, 1999	Overall sexual dysfunction	1410	DSM-IV	18-59	31
	Lacked interest in sex			18-29	14
				30-39	13
				40-49	15
				50-59	17
	Unable to achieve orgasm			18-29	7
				30-39	7
				40-49	9
				50-59	9
	Climax too early			18-29	30
				30-39	32
				40-49	28
				50-59	31
	Trouble maintaining or Achieving an erection			18-29	7
				30-39	9
				40-49	11
				50-59	18

CSFQ-14: Changes in Sexual Functioning Questionnaire short-form
DSM-IV: Diagnosis and Statistical Manual for Mental Disorder, 4th
PFSF: Profile of Female Sexual Function
IIEF: International Index of Erectile Function
BMSFI: Brief Male Sexual Function Inventory

Table 2. Characteristics of American studies of sexual dysfunction

	Problem or question	Sample size	Scale	Cohort age (year)	Prevalence (%)
Female					
Chen et al, 2003	Dyspareunia	112	Ad hoc questionnaire	40-55	44
Lau et al, 2005		3257	DSM-IV	18-59	
	Pain disorder				11.4
	Lubrication problems				23.7
	No orgasm				13.1
	No pleasure				16.2
Laumann et al, 2005		2106	Ad hoc questionnaire	40-80	
	Lack of sexual interest				39
	Inability to reach orgasm				36.7
	Orgasm too quickly				21.9
	Pain during sex				30.4
	Lubrication difficulties				36
Safarinejad 2006		2626	FSFI	20-60	
	Overall female sexual dysfunction				31.5
	Orgasmic disorder				
	Orgasmic disorder				37
	Arousal disorders				35
	Pain disorders				30
					26.7

Najafabady et al, 2011	Anorgasmia	1200	FSFI	20-40	26.3
Hisasue et al, 2005		5042	Ad hoc questionnaire		
	Orgasmic disorder			17-40	15.2
	Sexual desire disorder			17-40	32.2
	Arousal disorder			17-40	27.7
	Lubrication disorder			17-40	57.9
	Orgasmic disorder			40-70	29.7
	Sexual desire disorder			40-70	57.9
	Arousal disorder			40-70	12.5
	Lubrication disorder			40-70	51.2
Singh et al, 2009		149	FSFI	18+	
	Difficulties with desire				77.2
	Arousal disorder				91.3
	Lubrication problem				96.6
	Orgasmic disorder				86.6
	Pain disorder				64.4
Moreira et al, 2001		426	Ad hoc questionnaire	40-80	
	Lack of sexual pleasure				37
	Inability to reach orgasm				31
	Lubrication difficulties				29.4
	Pain during sex				28.1
	Lack of sexual interest				26.9
Sidi et al, 2007		230	FSFI	18-70	
	Lack of orgasms				59.1
	Low sexual arousal				60.9
	Lack of lubrication				50.4
	Sexual dissatisfaction				52.2
	Sexual pain				67.8
Sobhgol et al, 2007	Dyspareunia	319	Ad hoc questionnaire	15-49	54.5
Goshtasebi et al, 2009		1456	Ad hoc questionnaire	15+	
	Overall sexual dysfunction				52
	Desire difficulty				19.3
	Arousal difficulty				18.6
	Lubrication difficulty				11.9
	Orgasmic difficulty				21.3
	Pain difficulty				18.2
	Satisfaction difficulty				19.4
Male					
Lau et al, 2005		1516	DSM-IV	18-59	
	Pain disorder				3.4
	Erectile problems				9.6
	Premature orgasm				29.7
	No orgasm				7.2
Laumann et al, 2005	Lack of sexual interest	2701	Ad hoc questionnaire	40-80	23.8
	Inability to reach orgasm				19.1
	Early ejaculation				29.8
	Pain during sex				8.9
	Erectile difficulties				27.6
Nicolosi et al 2003	Erectile dysfunction	600	Ad hoc questionnaire	40-70	34

Junior et al, 2005	Early ejaculation Inability to reach orgasm Erectile difficulties Lack of sexual interest	471	Ad hoc questionnaire	40-80	30.3 14 13.1 11.2
Moreira et al, 2001	Early ejaculation Erectile difficulties Lack of sexual interest Inability to reach orgasm Sex not pleasurable	546	Ad hoc questionnaire	40-80	32.7 31.9 28.3 19.3 18.1
Kongkanand et al, 2000	Erectile difficulties	1259	Ad hoc questionnaire	40-70	37.5
Marumu et al, 2001	Erectile difficulties	1517	IIEF	23-29 30-39 40-49 50-59 60-69 70-79	19.2 2.3 9.5 15.7 34.4 53.4

DSM-IV: Diagnosis and Statistical Manual for Mental Disorder, 4th
FSFI: Female Sexual Function Index
IIEF: International Index of Erectile Function

Table 3. Characteristics of Asian studies of sexual dysfunction

	Problem or question	Sample size	Scale	Cohort age (year)	Prevalence (%)
Female					
Dennerstein et al, 2006	Hypoactive sexual desire disorder	2467	PFSF	50-70	12
Laumann et al, 2005	Lack of sexual interest Inability to reach orgasm Orgasm too quickly Pain during sex Lubrication difficulties	3494	Ad hoc questionnaire	40-80	27.6 20.9 9.6 10.4 17.2
Weiss et al, 2009	Arousal Disorder	1000	Ad hoc questionnaire	15-88	10.3
Ponholzer et al, 2004	desire disorders arousal disorders orgasmic problems Pain disorders	703	Ad hoc questionnaire	20-80	22 35 39 12.8
Hayes et al, 2008	hypoactive sexual desire disorder sexual arousal disorder (lubrication) orgasmic disorder dyspareunia	356	SFQ	20-70	16 7 8 1
Mercer et al, 2003	Lack of interest in sex	11161	ICD-10	16-44	40.6

	Unable to experience orgasm Premature orgasm Painful intercourse Trouble lubricating				14.4 1.3 11.8 9.2
Štulhofer et al, 2005	experienced sexual problems inhibited desire Inhibited arousal inhibited orgasm Dyspareunia	547	Ad hoc questionnaire	20-60	33.8 11.2 12.1 18.4 6.4
Dunn et al, 1998	Orgasmic Dysfunction Dyspareunia Vaginal Dryness problem with arousal inhibited enjoyment	979	Ad hoc questionnaire	18-75	27 18 18 17 18
Oksuz et al, 2006	overall sexual dysfunction desire problem arousal problem lubrication problem orgasm problem pain problem	518	FSFI	18-55	48.3 48.3 35.9 40.9 42.7 42.9
Danielsson et al, 2003	Dyspareunia	3017	Ad hoc questionnaire	20-60 20-29 30-39 40-49 50-60	9.3 13 10 8.6 6.5
TrÆen et al, 2010	Reduced sexual desire Problem achieving orgasm Genital pain	744	Ad hoc questionnaire	18-67	37 26 9
Male					
Braun et al, 2000	erectile dysfunction	4489	Ad hoc questionnaire	30-80 30-39 40-49 50-59 60-69 70-80	19.2 2.3 9.5 15.7 34.4 53.4
Laumann et al, 2005	Lack of sexual interest Inability to reach orgasm Early ejaculation Pain during sex Erectile difficulties	4311	Ad hoc questionnaire	40-80	12.7 10.6 21.1 3.6 13.1
Nicolosi et al 2003	erectile dysfunction	600	Ad hoc questionnaire	40-70	17
Mercer et al, 2003	Lack of interest in sex Unable to experience orgasm Premature orgasm	11161	ICD-10	16-44	17.1 5.3 11.7 17

	Painful intercourse Unable to achieve or maintain erection				5.8
Akkus et al, 2002	erectile dysfunction	1982	Ad hoc questionnaire	40+	69.2
Dunn et al, 1998	Difficulty getting erection Difficulty maintaining erection erectile dysfunction Premature ejaculation inhibited enjoyment	789	Ad hoc questionnaire	18-75	21 24 26 14 9
Giuliano et al, 2002	erectile dysfunction	1004	IIEF-5	40+ 40-49 50-59 60-69 ≥70	31.6 32.2 27 19.7 21
Parazzini et al, 2000	Erectile Dysfunction	2010	Ad hoc questionnaire	18+ 18-29 30-39 40-49 50-59 60-70 >70	12.8 2.8 1.9 4.8 15.7 26.8 48.3
Blanker, M et al, 2001	Erectile dysfunction Ejaculatory dysfunction	1688	ICS male sex questionnaire	50-54 55-59 60-64 65-69 70-78 50-54 55-59 60-64 65-69 70-78	3 5 11 19 26 3 5 11 21 35
TrÆen et al, 2010	Reduced sexual desire Problem achieving orgasm Genital pain	873	Ad hoc questionnaire	18-67	13 6 2
Martin-Morales et al, 2001	Erectile dysfunction	2476	IIEF Simple question	25-70	18.9 12.1

PFSF: Profile of Female Sexual Function
SFQ: Sexual Function Questionnaire
ICD-10: International Classification of Diagnosis-10
FSFI : Female Sexual Function Index
IIEF-5: International Index of Erectile Function-5
IIEF: International Index of Erectile Function

Table 4. Characteristics of European studies of sexual dysfunction

5. Conclusions

Existing epidemiologic data on sexual dysfunction support high prevalence of these problems worldwide. However, the data are limited and the prevalence data on male sexual dysfunction, except for ED, are too limited. Widely accepted definitions of disorders and scales are primary prerequisites to make prevalence comparisons possible and describe the severity of the problem.

6. Acknowledgement

Authors would like to thank Ms Zahra Sehat for searching and organizing papers.

7. References

Abdo, C. Oliveira, W. Moreira, E. Fittipaldi, J. 2004. Prevalence of sexual dysfunctions and correlated conditions in a sample of Brazilian women—results of the Brazilian study on sexual behavior (BSSB). International Journal of Impotence Research, 2004, 160–166.

Addis, I. Van Den Eeden, S. Wassel-Fyr, C. Vittinghoff, E. Brown, J. Thom, D. 2006. Sexual Activity and Function in Middle-Aged and Older Women. Obstet Gynecol. , 107, 4, 755–764.

Akkus, E. Kadioglo, A.Esen, A. Doran, A. Ergen, A. ans et. al. 2002. prevalence and correlate of erectile dysfunction in Turkey: a population based- study. Eropean Urology, 41,268-304.

Althof, S. 2006.Prevalence, Characteristics and Implications of Premature Ejaculation/Rapid Ejaculation. Journal of Urology, 175, 842-848.

Amidu, N. Owired, W. Gyasi-Sa rpong, C. Wood, E. Quaye, L. 2011. Sexual dysfunction among married couples living in Kumasi metropolis, Ghana. BMC Urology, 11, 3, 3-7.

Ansong, K. Lewis, C. Jenkins, P. Bell, J. 2000. Epidemiology of Erectile Dysfunction: A Community-based Study in Rural New York State. Ann Epidemiol ,10,293–296.

Bancroft, J. Loftus, J., Scott Long, J. 2003. Distress about Sex: A National Survey of Women in Heterosexual Relationships. Archives of Sexual Behavior, 32, 3, 193–208.

Blanker, M. Bosch, J. Grooeneveld, F. Bohnen, A. Thomas, A. Hop, W. 2001.Erectile and ejaculatory dysfunction in a community-based sample of men 50-78 years old: prevalence, concern, and relation to sexual activity. UROLOGY, 57,763-768.

Braun, M. Wassmer, G. Klotz, T. Reifenrath, B. Mathers, M. Engelmann, U. Epidemiology of erectile dysfunction: results of the `Cologne Male Survey'. 2000. International Journal of Impotence Research,12, 305-311.

Chen , O. 2003. Taneepanichskul, S. Prevalence of Dyspareunia in Healthy Thai Perimenopausal Women. Thai Journal of Obstetrics and Gynaecology, 15, 113-121.

Danielsson,I. berg, I. s Stenlund, H. Wikman, M. 2003. Prevalence and incidence of prolonged and severe dyspareunia in women: results from a population study. Scand J Public Health, 31, 113–118.

Dennerstein, L.Koochaki, P. Barton, I. Graziottin, A. 2006. Hypoactive sexual desire disorder in menopausal women: a survey of western European women. *The Journal of Sexual Medicine*, 3, 212-222.

Derby, C. Araujo, A Johannes, C. Feldman, H. McKinlay, J. 2000. Measurement of erectile dysfunction in population-based studies: the use of a single question self-assessment in the Massachusetts Male Aging Study. International Journal of Impotence Research,2000, 12, 197-204.

Dunn, k. Croft, P. Hackett, G. 1998.Sexual problem: a study of the prevalence and need for health care in the general population. Family Practice, 25,6, 519-524.

Elnashar, A. Ibrahim, M. EL-Deso ky, M. Ali, O. 2007. Mohamed Hassan, M. Female sexual dysf unction in Lower Egypt. BJOG, 114, 201 -206.

Giuliani, F. Cheveret- Measson, M. Tsatsaries, A. Reitz, C. Murino, M. thonneau, P. 2002. Prevalnce of erectile dysfunction in France: Result of an Epidemiologic survey of a reproductive sample of 1004 men. Eropean Urology, 42, 382-389.

Goshtasebi, A.Vahdaninia, M. Rahimi Foroshani, A. 2009. Prevalence and Potential Risk Factors of Female Sexual Difficulties: An Urban Iranian Population-Based Study. J Sex Med , 6, 2988–2996.

Hartmann U, Heiser K, Rüffer-Hesse C, Kloth G. Female sexual desire disorders: subtypes, classification, personality factors and new directions for treatment. 2002 World Journal of Urology; 20: 79-88.

Hassanin, I. Helmy, Y. Fathalla, M. Shahin, A. 2010. Prevalence and characteristics of female sexual dysfunction in a sample of women from Upper Egypt. International Journal of Gynecolo gy and Obstetrics 108, 219- 223.

Hayes RD, Dennerstein L, Bennett CM, Sidat M, Gurrin LC, and Fairley CK. Risk factors for female sexual dysfunction in the general population: Exploring factors associated with low sexual function and sexual distress. J Sex Med 2008;5:1681–1693.

Hisasue, S. kumamoto, Y. Sato, Y. Masumoori, N. Horit, H. and et al. 2005. Prevalence of female sexual dysfunction symptoms and its relationship to quality of life: A Japanese female cohort study. UROLOGY, 65,143–148.

Jonannes, c. Araujo, A. Feldman, H. Derby, C. 2000. Kleinnman, K. Mckinlay, J. Incidence of Erectile Dysfunction in Men 40 To 69 Years Old: Longitudinal Results from the Massachusetts Male Aging Study. The Journal of Urology, 163, 460 - 463.

Junior, E. Glasser, D. Santos, D. Gingell, C. 2005.Prevalence of sexual problems and related help-seeking behaviors among mature adults in Brazil: data from the Global Study of Sexual Attitudes and Behaviors. Sao Paulo Med J.123, 5, 234-41.

Kadri, K. Alami, M. Tahiri, M. 2002, Sexual dysfunction in women: population based epidemiological study. Arch Womens Ment Health , 5,59–63.

Kinsey AC, Pomeroy WB, Martin CE and Gebhard PH. Sexual Behavior in the Human Female. W. B. Saunders & Co. Philadelphia 1953.

Kongkanand, A. 2000. Prevalence of erectile dysfunction in Thailand. International Journal of Andrology, 23, 2, 77-80.

Lau, J. Kim JH. Tsui, H-Y. 2005. Prevalence of male and female sexual problems, perceptions related to sex and association with quality of life in a Chinese population: a population-based study. International Journal of Impotence Research, 17, 494–505.

Laumann, E. Das, A. Waite, L. 2008. Sexual Dysfunction among Older Adults: Prevalence and Risk Factors from a Nationally Representative U.S. Probability Sample of Men and Women 57–85 Years of Age. J SexMed ,5, 10, 2300–2311.

Laumann, E. Paik, A. Rosen, R.1999. Sexual Dysfunction in the United States Prevalence and Predictors. JAMA, 2, 81:537-544.

Laumann, EO. Nicolosi, A. Glasser, DB. Paik, A. Gingell, C. Moreira, E. Wang, T. 2005. Sexual problems among women and men aged 40–80 y: prevalence and correlates identified in the Global Study of Sexual Attitudes and Behaviors. International Journal of Impotence Research,17, 39–57.

Lindau, s. Schumm, P. Laumann, O. Levinson, W. O'Muircheartaigh, C. Waite, L. 2007. A Study of Sexuality and Health among Older Adults in the United States.. N Engl J Med, 357, 22-34.

Marumu, K. Nakashima, J. Murai, M.2001. Age related prevalence of erectile dysfunction in Japan. Assessment by the international index of erectile dysfunction. International Journal of Urology, 8, 53-59.

Mercer, C. Fenton, K. Johnson, A. Wellings, K. Macdowall, W. McManus, S. Nanchahal, K. Erens, B. 2003.Sexual function problems and help seeking behavior in Britain: national probability sample survey. BMJ. 327, 23, 426-427.

Martin-Morales A, Sanchez-Cruz JJ, Saenz de Tejada I, Rodriguez-Vela L, Jimenez-Cruz JF, Burgos-Rodriguez R. 2001. Prevalence and independent risk factors for erectile dysfunction in Spain: results of the Epidemiologia de la Disfuncion Erectil Masculina Study. Journal of urology,166,569-74.

Moreira, E. Adbo, C. Torres, E. Lobo, C. Fittipaldi, N.2001. prevalence and correlates of erectile dysfunction: result of the Brazilian study of sexual behavior. UROLOGY, 58, 583–588.

Najafabady MT, Salmani Z, Abedi P. 2011. Prevalence and related factors for anorgasmia among reproductive aged women in Hesarak, Iran. Clinics (Sao Paulo); 66, 83-6.

Nicolosi, A. Morejra, E. Shirai, M. Tambi, M. Glasser, D. 2003.Epidemiology of erectile dysfunction in four countries: cross-national study of the prevalence and correlates of erectile dysfunction. J of Urology, 61,1, 201-206.

Oksuz, E. Malhan, S. 2006. Prevalence and Risk Factors for Female Sexual Dysfunction in Turkish Women. THE JOURNAL OF UROLOGY, 175, 654-658.

Parazzini F, Menchini Fabris F, Bortolotti A, Calabrò A, Chatenoud L, Colli E, Landoni M, Lavezzari M, Turchi P, Sessa A, Mirone V. 2000. Frequency and determinants of erectile dysfunction in Italy. Eur Urol;37:43-9.

Prins, J. Blanker, MH. Bohnen, AM. Thomas, S. Bosch, J. 2002. Prevalence of erectile dysfunction: a systematic review of population-based studies. *International Journal of Impotence Research*, 14, 422–432.

Ponholzera, A.Roehlicha, M. Racza, U. Temmla, C. Madersbacher, S. 2005. Female Sexual Dysfunction in a HealthyAustrian Cohort: Prevalence and Risk Factors. European Urology, 47, 366–375.

Safarinejad, MR. 2006. Female sexual dysfunction in a population-based study in Iran: prevalence and associated risk factors. International Journal of Impotence Research, 18, 382–395

Saigal, C. Wessells, H. Pace, J. Schonlau, M.Wilt, T. 2006. Predictors and Prevalence of Erectile Dysfunction in a Racially Diverse Population. Arch Intern Med,166,207-212.

Seyam, R. Albakry, A.Ghobish, A. Arif, H. Dandash, K. Rashwan, H. 2003.Prevalence of erectile dysfunction and its correlates in Egypt: a community-based study. International Journal of Impotence Research, 15, 237–245.

Shifren, J. Monz, B. Russo, P. Segreti, A. Johannes, C. 2008. Sexual Problems and Distress in United States Women: Prevalence and Correlates. Obstet Gynecol, 112, 970–8.

Sidi, H. Puteh, S.Abdullah, N. Midin, M. 2007. The Prevalence of Sexual Dysfunction and Potential Risk Factors That May Impair Sexual Function in Malaysian Women. J Sex Med, 4, 311-321.

Simons, J. Carey, M.2001. Prevalence of Sexual Dysfunctions: Results from a Decade of Research. Arch Sex Behav, 30, 2, 177-219.

Singh, j. Tharyan, P. Kekre, N. Singh, G. Gopalakrishnan, G. 2009. Prevalence and risk factors for female sexual dysfunction in women attending a medical clinic in south India. Journal of Post Gratuate Medicine, 55, 2, 113-120.

Sobhgol, S.Mohammad Alizadeli Charndabee, S. 2007. Rate and related factors of dyspareunia in reproductive age women: a cross-sectional study. International Journal of Impotence Research,19, 88-94.

Štulhofer,A. Gregurovię , M. Pikię, A. Galię, A. 2005. Sexual Problems o f Urban Women in Croatia: Prevalence and Correlates in a Community Sample. Croat Med J, 46, 1,45-51.

Tiefer, L. 2001. A new view of women's sexual problem: why new? why now?. J Sex Research, 38, 89-96.

TrÆen, B. Stigun, H. 2010. Sexual problems in 18-67-year-old Norwegians. Scandinavian Journal of Public Health, 38, 445-456.

Tsai, T. Yeh, C. Hwang, T. 2011. Female Sexual Dysfunction: Physiology, Epidemiology, Classification, Evaluation and Treatment. Urol Sci, 22, 1, 7–13.

Weiss, P. Brody, S. 2009. Female Sexual Arousal Disorder with and without a Distress Criterion: Prevalence and Correlates in a Representative Czech Sample. J Sex Med, 6, 3385-3394.

West, S. D'Aloisio, A. Agans, R. Kalsbeek, W. Borisov, N. Thorp, J. 2008. Prevalence of Low Sexual Desire and Hypoactive Sexual Desire Disorder in a Nationally Representative Sample of US Women. Arch Intern Med, 168, 13,1441-1449.

Part 2

Sexual Dysfunction in Special Conditions

2

Maintenance Therapy and Sexual Behavior

Salvatore Giacomuzzi[1,2], Klaus Garber[3],
Alessandra Farneti[3] and Yvonne Riemer[4]
[1]*Free University of Bolzano,*
[2]*University of Innsbruck, Institute of Psychology,*
[3]*UMIT - The private University for Health Sciences, Medical Informatics and Technology,*
[4]*University Hospital Innsbruck; Department for Psychiatry and Psychotherapy,*
[1]*Italy*
[2,3,4]*Austria*

1. Introduction

Today, the term "human sexual behavior" sounds familiar and is so widely used that it may be hard to imagine a time when it was unknown (Haeberle, 1981; 1983). However, the realization that people have always done certain things does not necessarily allow us to conclude that they have always thought of them the same way.

Linguists also know that seemingly simple words often have no exact equivalents in other languages and that, as the years go by, they may very well change their meaning (Haeberle, 1981; 1983).

Obviously, the distinction between physical and psychological causes of sexual inadequacy is, to a certain extent, arbitrary, since body and mind are so closely interrelated that a sharp dividing line between them cannot be drawn. Some men and women are restricted in their sexual expression by physical malformations, handicaps, diseases, or injuries.

However, there are also physically healthy individuals who cannot fully enjoy sexual intercourse because their sexual responses have become weakened, inhibited, or even completely blocked for psychological reasons. Today, such a person is usually said to suffer from "sexual inadequacy" or "sexual dysfunction" (Haeberle, 1981; 1983).

Very few people enjoy perfect health throughout their lives. Sooner or later, most of us find ourselves in need of medical attention, if only temporarily. Of course, many of the serious diseases that plague and cripple mankind also have a damaging effect on sexual abilities. Certain illnesses can affect a person's responses or weaken the body to a point where sexual intercourse becomes difficult or impossible.

Usually in such cases, the sexual difficulties are only the by-product of a general infirmity and therefore receive only minor attention (Haeberle, 1981; 1983).

There are, however, certain physical disorders and diseases that affect human sexual activity and procreation directly, such as for example addiction.

Opioid maintenance treatment is the most widespread and well-researched treatment modality for opioid dependence (Giacomuzzi, 2008; 2011; Brown & Zueldorff 2007). Methadone, slow-release oral morphine and buprenorphine are currently the most commonly used pharmacotherapeutic agents.

Maintenance treatment has become a major intervention in the care and treatment of drug dependence in Europe. But still little is known about sexual behavior and sexual dysfunction especially under maintenance treatment.
A greater understanding of sexual behaviour in different maintenance treatment contexts has important consequences for the design and evaluation of substitution programs in opioid therapy.
Sexual dysfunction has been reported as an adverse effect of opioids including methadone and buprenorphine maintenance treatment.
In recognition of this, this chapter also aims to present specific problems and facts regarding this issue. Furthermore, the chapter presents own results regarding sexual behaviour and dysfunction prevalence within maintenance treatment. This chapter therefore provides some basic information about the main physical illnesses and impairments which can interfere with human sexual functioning regarding addiction.

2. Addiction and maintenance treatment

Opioids are commonly prescribed because of their effective analgesic, or pain-relieving, properties. Medications that fall within this class - referred to as prescription narcotics - include morphine, codeine, oxycodone (e.g., OxyContin, Percodan, Percocet), and related drugs.
Morphine, for example, is often used before and after surgical procedures to alleviate severe pain. Codeine, on the other hand, is often prescribed for mild pain.
In addition to their pain-relieving properties, some of these drugs - codeine and diphenoxylate (Lomotil), for example - can be used to relieve coughs and diarrhea (National Institute on Drug Abuse, 2011).
Opioids act on the brain and body by attaching to specific proteins called opioid receptors, which are found in the brain, spinal cord, and gastrointestinal tract.
When these drugs attach to certain opioid receptors, they can block the perception of pain. Opioids can produce drowsiness, nausea, constipation, and, depending upon the amount of drug taken, depress respiration. Opioid drugs also can induce euphoria by affecting the brain regions that mediate what we perceive as pleasure. This feeling is often intensified for those who abuse opioids, when administered by routes other than those recommended. For example, OxyContin is often snorted or injected to enhance its euphoric effects, while at the same time increasing the risk of serious medical consequences, such as opioids overdose.
Many studies have shown that the properly managed, short-term medical use of opioid analgesic drugs is safe and rarely causes addiction - defined as the compulsive and uncontrollable use of drugs despite adverse consequences - or dependence, which occurs when the body adapts to the presence of a drug, and often results in withdrawal symptoms when that drug is reduced or stopped.
Withdrawal symptoms include restlessness, muscle and bone pain, insomnia, diarrhea, vomiting, cold flashes with goose bumps ("cold turkey"), and involuntary leg movements.
Taking a large single dose of an opioid could cause severe respiratory depression that can lead to death (National Institute on Drug Abuse, 2011).
Long-term use of opioids can lead to physical dependence and addiction.
Addiction continues to be referred to by terms such as drug dependence and psychological dependence (Federation of State Medical Boards of the United States, 1998).

The traditional distinction between addiction and habituation centers on the ability of a drug to produce tolerance and physical dependence. Tolerance is a physiological phenomenon that requires the individual to use more and more of the drug in repeated efforts to achieve the same effect.

Physical dependence manifests itself through the signs and symptoms of abstinence when the drug is withdrawn. A classic feature of physical dependence is the abstinence or withdrawal syndrome. If the addict is abruptly deprived of a drug upon which the body has physical dependence, there will ensue a set of reactions, the intensity of which will depend on the amount and length of time that the drug has been used.

Physical dependence and tolerance are normal physiological consequences of extended opioid therapy for pain and should not be considered addiction (American Academy of Pain Medicine and the American Pain Society, 1997; Commission of Public Records, 2003).

Addiction is currently also defined as a form of behavior through which an individual has impaired control with harmful consequences. Thus, individuals who recognize that their behavior is harming them or those they care about find themselves unable to stop engaging in the behavior when they try to do so (Giacomuzzi, 2008).

The severity of the medical, psychological and social harm that can be caused by addiction, together with the fact that it violates the individual's freedom of choice, means that it is appropriate to consider it to be a disorder of motivation.

A very commonly used reference text from the American Psychiatric Association - the Diagnostic and Statistical Manual of Mental Disorders - does not use the term addiction at all; rather, it uses substance dependence. And, to be more precise, the particular drug involved is specified: e.g., heroin dependence, alcohol dependence, etc.

Although other forms of treatment for opioid dependence continue to be explored, methadone maintenance treatment remains the most widely used form of treatment for people who are dependent on opioids.

Methadone maintenance treatment is a key component of a comprehensive treatment and prevention strategy to address opioid dependence and its consequences (Giacomuzzi et al., 2003; 2008; 2009).

Methadone was originally developed in Germany as a substitute analgesic for morphine. World War II brought the formula to the attention of North American researchers, who subsequently discovered that methadone could be used to treat heroin withdrawal symptoms in 1964 as a medical response to the post-World War II heroin epidemic in New York City (Giacomuzzi, 2008).

The principal effects of methadone maintenance are to relieve narcotic craving, suppress the abstinence syndrome, and block the euphoric effects associated with heroin. Methadone works by alleviating the symptoms of opioid withdrawal. A stable and sufficient blood level of methadone stems the chronic craving for opioids.

Since methadone is a much longer acting drug than some other opioids, such as heroin, one oral dose daily prevents the onset of opioid withdrawal symptoms - including anxiety, restlessness, runny nose, tearing, nausea and vomiting - for 24 hours or longer. Methadone diminishes the euphoric effects of other opioids (cross tolerance), without necessarily causing euphoria, sedation or analgesia.

This means that self-administered illicit opioids will not lead to euphoria, making it less likely that clients/patients will either use illicit opioids or overdose (Giacomuzzi, 2008).

Methadone maintenance treatment has been demonstrated to be an effective treatment for opioid addiction and curbs the incidence thereof. Although methadone maintenance

treatment has been successful, it is associated with a number of problems. Up to 50% of methadone patients withdraw from treatment in the first 6 months. Daily dosing can be a burden for treatment facilities, some of which provide doses to over 900 patients a day. Patients prefer take-home doses, but they are often associated with diversion. Therefore, nowadays methadone cannot be regarded as the golden standard for all addicted persons.
There are a number of alternatives to methadone as a maintenance agent in the management of opioid dependence.
The most promising of these involve pharmacotherapies which treat patients with a pharmaceutical grade opioid which has a longer duration of action than methadone. These include the opioid partial agonist buprenorphine and the full agonist levo-alpha-acetylmethadol (LAAM) (Giacomuzzi, 2008).

2.1 Buprenorphine maintenance treatment

Buprenorphine is a potent synthetic opioid analgesic initially used for the management of acute pain. Pharmacologically, buprenorphine causes morphine-like subjective effects and produces cross-tolerance to other opioids. Unlike methadone and heroin (which are full agonists), buprenorphine is a partial agonist and exerts weaker opioid effects at opioid receptor sites.
This partial agonist action appears to make buprenorphine safer in overdose. Other benefits of buprenorphine may include an easier withdrawal phase and, because of the longer duration of action, the option of alternate day dosing (Giacomuzzi et al., 2005; 2008).
It was during the initial development of buprenorphine as an analgesic in the 1970s that its potential utility as a substitution agent in the treatment of opioid dependence was recognised. Early work using buprenorphine administered subcutaneously characterised it as an opioid with low physical dependence liability with a minimal withdrawal syndrome.
Subsequently, others provided evidence that buprenorphine does produce a mild to moderate mu-agonist withdrawal syndrome. It was thought that at doses somewhat greater than those used for analgesia, it could be used in the treatment of opioid dependence. Buprenorphine also has also some advantages over methadone. As mentioned earlier, buprenorphine has a ceiling level on agonist activity, limiting adverse reactions at very high doses. Some study results suggest that a twice-weekly dosing regimen may also be possible (Petry et al., 2001).
Evidence on the efficacy of buprenorphine has come from placebo-controlled trials, fixed dosing studies of buprenorphine versus methadone maintenance treatment and variable dosing studies of buprenorphine versus methadone maintenance treatment (Giacomuzzi, 2008). Some of the fixed dose studies showed no difference in efficacy, whereas others showed superiority for methadone and yet others showed the opposite pattern.
The investigators of these fixed dose studies frequently concluded that the doses of buprenorphine or methadone chosen were too low or that poor induction regimes led to poor retention. A series of variable (or flexible) dose studies have been conducted and show essentially equivalent results for the two drugs.
The implication of the results of a meta-analytic review conducted and reported by Mattick et al. (2004) is clear for clinical practice. The authors conclude that buprenorphine is an effective treatment for heroin use in a maintenance therapy approach.
A meta-analysis comparing buprenorphine to methadone for treatment of opioid dependence found that subjects who received 8-12 mg/d buprenorphine had 1.26 times the

relative risk of discontinuing treatment than subjects receiving 50-80 mg/d methadone. In this meta-analysis, buprenorphine was more effective than 20-35 mg/d methadone.

These studies also found that the difference in the effectiveness of buprenorphine and methadone may be statistically significant, but the difference was small compared to the wide variance in outcomes achieved in different methadone treatment programmes (Giacomuzzi, 2008; 2009).

Randomized, controlled studies of up to 6 months' duration compared sublingual buprenorphine with methadone in opioid dependent patients. These generally demonstrated comparable efficacy with buprenorphine 8-12mg/d and methadone 30-90mg/d in promoting retention in treatment and reducing illicit opioid.

Nevertheless, it is buprenorphine that has gained more and more importance in addiction treatment because the correlation between dose and therapeutic effects is not linear, indicating a ceiling on the effects in patients due to its opioid agonistic-antagonistic characteristics.

Buprenorphine is therefore a relatively safe substance, and its effectiveness in maintenance therapy has been proved in many studies. It has been used in Austria as a substitution drug since 1999.

Further research is needed to determine whether buprenorphine treatment is more effective than methadone in particular settings or in particular subgroups of patients.

It should be noted that, in an effort to prevent injection of the drug, the Buprenorphine/Naloxone - Sublingual Suboxone® formulation includes naloxone in addition to buprenorphine. Until now, these efforts have turned out to be less fruitful and the acceptance of this new group of preparations (Suboxone®) appears to have decreased in contrast to classical buprenorphine (Subutex®).

However, reasons which lower the acceptance on the part of the clients yet are not fully understood (Giacomuzzi et al., 2011).

2.2 Slow-release oral morphine maintenance treatment

Nowadays, apart from methadone and sublingual buprenorphine, another substitution medication is prescribed for opioid treatment, such as long-acting morphine (retarded or slow-release oral morphine).

Slow-release oral morphine was established in 1998 for substitution, which gives Austria an exceptional position in opioid addiction treatment compared to other European countries (Giacomuzzi, 2008).

Although slow-release oral morphine is used in Austria as an alternative to methadone or buprenorphine for maintenance treatment of opioid dependence, quantitative descriptions of patient outcomes have yet to be reported.

Slow-release oral morphine is an opioid agonist with a 12–24 hour duration of action. It is indicated for use as a maintenance treatment. The slow-release form overcomes many of the disadvantages of the short-acting nature of morphine, so theoretically it should have the same treatment effects as methadone, without some of methadone's disadvantages. Therefore, slow-release oral morphine has been proposed as an alternative maintenance pharmacotherapy to methadone or sublingual buprenorphine for treatment of opioid dependence.

There have been several studies on slow-release oral morphine for maintenance therapy Giacomuzzi, 2008). Morphine is not usually administered at our clinic to children under the age of 18 years, in respiratory depressions and in the presence of acute alcoholism (Giacomuzzi, 2008). Further research is needed to determine whether slow-release oral morphine treatment is more effective than methadone or buprenorphine in particular settings or in particular subgroups of patients.

3. Effects of opioid maintenance treatment on sexual dysfunctions

Consideration of side effects of opioid pharmacotherapies like cognitive impairment or sexual dysfunction is important. Especially sexual dysfunction, besides creating difficulty in intimate relationships, has the potential to lead to decreased compliance with therapy and to interfere with the known benefits of opioid maintenance treatment.
While the impact of sexual dysfunction upon treatment compliance has scarcely been studied in opioid maintenance treatment-receiving samples, sexual dysfunction has been shown to interfere with therapeutic compliance among subjects with depression, HIV, and hypertension (Brown & Zueldorff, 2007; Giacomuzzi 2008).

3.1 Sexual dysfunction among men and woman

Sexual dysfunction among men on opioid maintenance treatment appears to be related to lower-than-normal serum levels of testosterone. The association between opioids and low serum testosterone levels may occur through a variety of mechanisms (Brown & Zueldorff, 2007). Opioids may also act directly upon testicular tissue to suppress normal testosterone production.
Research regarding sexual dysfunction among females on opioid maintenance treatment is more scant. Sexual dysfunction among women on opioid maintenance treatment appears to be primarily related to interference with the normal cyclic production, possibly due to elevated production of prolactin mechanisms (Brown & Zueldorff, 2007).
This process interferes both with hormones necessary for the maintenance of a normal menstrual cycle (estrogen, progesterone) and for normal libido (androgens). Interference with these sex hormones is thought to lead to the common signs and symptoms of sexual dysfunction and hormonal dysregulation, and among women on opioid maintenance treatment, depressed libido and oligomenorrhea or amenorrhea mechanisms (Brown & Zueldorff, 2007).
Especially literature regarding sexual dysfunction in female subjects on opioid maintenance treatment is also very scant. Studies have indicated that 50% of women switching from heroin to methadone experienced an improvement in sexual function.
Methadone was shown to depress serum testosterone levels in female subjects in one study. This depression of testosterone in women was also associated with increases in serum prolactin (Brown & Zueldorff, 2007).
Nearly 50% of women experience menstrual irregularity while on methadone maintenance. The effect appears to be dose-related, and appears to decline over time, with the potential for resumption of normal menses without alteration of methadone dosing (Brown & Zueldorff, 2007).
While it is clear that impaired androgen production is closely and directly associated with sexual dysfunction in males, the relationship within females is more complicated and less clear (Brown & Zueldorff, 2007; Giacomuzzi, 2009).
The normal mid-cycle rise in serum androgens in women has not been strongly related to sex drive. Transdermal replacement of lower-than-normal serum androgens in female

subjects, however, has been shown to result in improvements in mood and libido. Additionally, when given testosterone supplementation, women with normal levels of serum testosterone have demonstrated an increased sexual response mechanism (Brown & Zueldorff, 2007).

Studies have demonstrated higher rates of sexual dysfunction in methadone-maintained groups than in the general population. Estimates of prevalence, however, vary significantly between 30-100%.

Additionally, the prevalence of specific types of sexual dysfunction (libido, erectile, and orgasm dysfunction) has poorly been examined in detail (Brown & Zueldorff, 2007; Giacomuzzi, 2009).

In one of the first studies to examine particular types of sexual dysfunction in a methadone maintained sample, Teusch et al. (1995) found men maintained on methadone to report reduced libido and orgasm dysfunction more frequently than controls.

Similar to earlier studies, however, the severity of dysfunction and methadone dose were unrelated.

Mendelson et al conducted a prospective study of the effect of acetylmethadol administration on serum testosterone levels in 13 men with opioid dependence which yielded significant results. A statistically and biologically significant decrease in serum testosterone was found 7-9 hours after acetylmethadol administration. Testosterone levels attained normal levels 48 hours after drug administration.

Mendelson also conducted some of the earliest work demonstrating a relationship between methadone dose and serum testosterone concentration. When the sample (n =38) was dichotomized into groups receiving lower dose (10-60 mg) and higher dose (80-150 mg) methadone, the men receiving higher daily doses of methadone were found to be more likely to have abnormally low serum testosterone.

As further evidence of an inverse relationship between methadone dose and serum testosterone levels in this study, reductions in methadone dose were associated with recovery of testosterone levels.

Mendelson et al found similar results in a sample of 10 men administered heroin in a controlled setting for 7 days and then detoxified using methadone at a starting dose of 35 mg. Again, abnormally low serum testosterone levels found during and after the period of heroin administration were found to recover to baseline after methadone detoxification.

3.2 Erectile dysfunctions

Erectile dysfunction (ED) more commonly has an organic or iatrogenic etiology. A variety of systemic illnesses are associated with ED. These include chronic liver disease, renal failure, arteriosclerotic cardiovascular disease, diabetes mellitus, chronic obstructive pulmonary disease, and malignancy. Spinal trauma and genitourinary surgery are of potential etiologic importance in ED, as well.

Though rarer, congenital and other anatomic genitourinary anomalies (e.g. Peyronie's Disease, phimosis, post-traumatic aneurysm) should also be considered (Brown & Zueldorff, 2007).

Medications commonly associated with ED include antihypertensives, psychotropic agents, and medications with anticholinergic effects.

Smoking, for example, is strongly associated with ED. The relative risk for ED increases by 1.31 for every 10 pack-years of smoking.

Though organic factors commonly cause ED, mental and emotional health issues may be significant contributors, as well. Depressive symptoms have been most strongly associated with ED, with 90% of men with severe depression reporting ED in one study. Association with anxiety disorders has also been reported (Brown & Zueldorff, 2007).
Several previous studies have demonstrated that erectile dysfunction (ED) is common among heroin users and people undergoing treatment for heroin addiction. Estimates of the prevalence of ED in methadone-maintained patients vary widely: 16% (8 cases/50 subjects), 23%.
Many patients with ED fail to mention ED to clinicians and counsellors and many clinicians and counsellors feel uncomfortable and embarrassed about dealing with sexual problems.
Nevertheless, the assessment of ED in these patients may be quite important. Identification and management of ED problems can improve adherence to treatment, the effectiveness of which, as is well-known, is associated with high doses and long treatment duration.
It is hard to establish the relative importance of possible causes of ED among opioid users.
Many drugs commonly prescribed for co-morbid conditions among drug users (antidepressants, antipsychotics, sedatives, anxiolytics, anticholinergics, etc.) can negatively affect sexual performance (Brown & Zueldorff, 2007).
Low testosterone levels may be a relevant cause of ED among opioid users, although no conclusive results have been reached. Two physiological mechanisms are thought to be responsible for the reported ED associated with opioid use.
The first is the inhibition of the production of gonadotropin-releasing hormone, decreasing the release of the luteinizing hormone (LH) and therefore reducing the production of testosterone.
Opioids can also cause hyperprolactinemia, which produces negative feedback on the release of LH and consequently on the secretion of testosterone.
However, existing studies involve few patients, and no correlation between duration of methadone treatment and testosterone blood levels has been found. Moreover, in the general population, endocrinal causes are responsible only in a small number of cases of ED (Brown & Zueldorff, 2007).
A study by Quaglio et al. (2008) included 201 males; subjects were 18–47 years old (mean = 31, S.D. = 6.0). Eighty-five patients (42%) were on methadone maintenance with a median dose of 40 mg/day (min 10, max 180 mg, 5% above 100 mg/day).
One hundred sixteen patients (58%) were on buprenorphine maintenance with a median dose of 6 mg/day (min 1, max 24, slightly more than 10% had dosages over 12 mg/day). As reported, subjects in methadone and buprenorphine treatment had similar socio-demographic characteristics (the hypothesis of distribution homogeneity was not rejected for almost all study variables).
Fifty-nine percent reported no depression, 24% reported mild depression, 12% moderate and 4% serious depression.
In all, 67 patients declared they did not have a steady sexual partner: consequently, the characteristics of steady sexual partners are based on data from 134 subjects. These partners were, on average, 3.4 years (S.D. = 6.3) younger than the index subjects, 68% of the partners were employed, 40% had no more than 8 years of education, and 14% of the partners had used heroin.
In the study of Quaglio et al. (2008), very substantial rates of ED were found: 19%of the patients reported severe ED and another 23%reported mild to moderate ED.

The percentage of patients reporting ED is moderately higher than the percentages reporting ED in previous studies of methadone patients (Brown et al., 2004; Hanbury et al., 1977; Teusch et al., 1995; Cushman, 1972).

The majority of previous studies of ED among drug users have used nonvalidated questionnaires, so caution should be exercised when comparing these earlier study findings to the present results.

Nevertheless, all the surveys by Quaglio et al. (2008) indicate high rates of ED among methadone/buprenorphine patients. However, the age of the subjects in this study ranged from 18 to 47, with a mean age of 31 where 42% reported ED, while in a general population study of more than 2000 Italian males, only 2% in the age group 18–39 reported ED.

In a study by Quaglio et al. (2008), the univariate analysis showed a significant association between treatment and ED, with buprenorphine patients reporting less ED than methadone patients, but this was not confirmed by the multivariate analysis.

Quaglio et al. (2008) did not find any significant association between either methadone dose or buprenorphine dose and ED, or with reported duration of either methadone or buprenorphine treatment and ED.

Thus, these data by Quaglio et al. (2008) do not suggest that changing from one medication to the other, or modest changes in the dosage level of either medication, would be effective in reducing ED.

The association between depression and ED is well established in literature and the causal relationship is probably bidirectional, i.e. ED may be a consequence of depression and depression may follow ED. About 1/3 of depressed untreated patients report reduced libido, delayed ejaculation, anorgasm or ED.

Comorbidity of mood disorders and opioid dependence has also been frequently observed. Seventeen per cent of our patients suffered from depression, while only 6% were on anti-depression treatment, and there was no association between receiving or not receiving treatment and ED. The routine assessment of patients in opioid agonist treatment should include a careful evaluation of depression and, when clinically indicated, vigorous treatment.

Three aspects of social/sexual relationships were associated with ED in the study of Quaglio et al. (2008).

Living with a sexual partner (compared to living with parents) was associated with a lower likelihood of ED. Having ED may reduce one's ability to develop and maintain a sufficiently strong sexual relationship to lead to the partners living together. Lack of a steady partner may also contribute to ED.

Quaglio et al. (2008) also found that living with a sexual partner who has a history of heroin use was associated with current ED in these patients.

The association in the study of Quaglio et al. (2008) was very strong, with an adjusted odds ratio of 5.84, which reflects the relevant decrement of the median ED score from 27 in the patients with a non-heroin user partner to 21 in those with a heroin-user partner. Another study observed that when both members of a couple are strongly addicted to heroin, they almost always lose interest in sex.

All the patients in this study, however, had entered drug abuse treatment in order to reduce their heroin use, and it was assumed that interest in sex would return during treatment. There are (at least) two interesting mechanisms in this strong association.

Difficulties in the relationship between two people with histories of heroin abuse may lead to ED, and/or males with a pre-disposition to ED may selectively seek out females who use heroin as sexual partners.

In this study, Quaglio et al. (2008) found a high rate of ED among Italian methadone and buprenorphine patients—18% had severe ED and 24% had mild to moderate ED. Both psychological factors (depression) and social factors (living situation, lack of steady partner, whether partner had a history of heroin use) were associated with ED.
The cross-sectional design of the study precludes determining whether these associations represented mere correlations without causal relationships, whether the factors were causes of ED, or whether ED was the cause of the factors, or some combination of all of these possibilities.
It is also important to note that no data was available on ED among these patients prior to their entry into methadone or buprenorphine treatment, either during periods of intense heroin use or during periods of abstinence from heroin.
There was also no data on the current use of other drugs which might influence the sexual functioning of the patients.
The strengths of the study of Quaglio et al. (2008) include a large sample of patients, its multicentral nature and the identification of predictors for diagnosis.
In addition, their paper presents ED for a large cohort of patients in buprenorphine treatment.
Quaglio et al. (2008) conclude that ED is likely to be an important problem for many males in methadone and buprenorphine treatment, and good addiction treatment will need to address this issue. Androgen replacement and pharmacological treatment may be effective approaches for these patients.
Counselling of couples may also be useful. In our view, taking patients off methadone or buprenorphine, with the high risk of relapse to intensive heroin use, would not be suitable.

Specific study findings on buprenorphine

Studies comparing buprenorphine to the more commonly used methadone have found that rates of success in treatment are similar and that buprenorphine may result in fewer adverse effects. However, only a few studies to date have examined the prevalence of sexual dysfunction in particular among patients treated with buprenorphine and it is important that the influence of buprenorphine on ED be investigated further in the near future (Brown & Zueldorff, 2007; Giacomuzzi 2008; 2009).
One previous study found that buprenorphine has fewer negative effects on male sexual performance than methadone (Bliesener et al., 2005). This study, however, included only a small number of subjects, 17 patients in buprenorphine and 37 in methadone treatment.
In 2005, Bliesener and colleagues examined 17 male patients maintained on buprenorphine and 37 male patients maintained on methadone. Patients self-reported effects on libido and potency, and total and free testosterone, estradiol, and prolactin were assayed. Blood samples from 51 male volunteers were used as a control group for the hormone analyses. Twenty-three percent of patients in the buprenorphine group reported a decrease in libido, compared to 83% in the methadone group. Twelve percent reported reduced potency, compared to 72% in the methadone group.
Other forms of sexual dysfunction, such as orgasm dysfunction, were not examined in this study.
The Bliesener study also found that patients treated with buprenorphine had significantly higher mean levels of total (5.1 ± 1.2 ng/mL) and free (17.1 ± 4.8 pg/mL) testosterone than patients treated with methadone (2.8 ± 1.2 ng/mL and 7.8 ± 2.9 pg/mL, respectively), and

that in fact mean total testosterone levels of those patients being treated with buprenorphine did not significantly differ from levels in the healthy control group sample (4.9 ± 1.3 ng/mL).

Mean levels of prolactin were significantly higher in the methadone group (8.7 ± 8.3 ng/mL) than in the buprenorphine group (5.0 ± 2.0 ng/mL), though all groups were in the normal range. There were no other significant differences found in the hormonal analysis.

In an examination of BDI scores collected in the same study, mean scores of the opioid therapy groups were not found to differ significantly from one another.

This lack of difference, as well as a lack of significant difference in age, medical status, length of addiction, concurrent medications, or frequency of illicit opioid use led the authors to conclude that it was most likely the treatment drug rather than other variables that contributed to the differences between therapy groups in hormone levels and reports of sexual dysfunction.

The aim of our own examination was to determine which substitution agent seemed most suitable as a substitution drug for narcotic-addicted men and women in relation to both sexuality and relationship quality. In particular, the examination of female sexuality amongst women administered substitutes presented a considerable challenge, both in psychological and medical terms.

As part of sex research by Büsing, Hoppe und Liedtke in 2000, an examination of 'Sexual satisfaction amongst women - survey development and results' was carried out. The subject of this study focussed on the conception, creation and execution of a survey to determine the sexual satisfaction of women. As basic data, the survey considered the frequency and duration of sexual activity, satisfaction with the frequency and duration of the activity and desired sexual behavior. In the first study, 112 heterosexual women between the ages of 20-48 were interviewed. On the one hand, the results reveal the importance of the orgasm experience, which is emphasised through the high rate of desire concerning coital orgasm. On the other hand, half of the women who participated in the study did not state orgasm as their favourite part of sex. 37% of the women state that the emotional and physical closeness to their partner is more important than climaxing. In between-group comparison, sexual satisfaction above all correlates with the degree of autonomy within the relationship, satisfaction of communicative desires within the relationship and the need for affection. (Büsing et al. 2000)

This study shows that assessing sexual satisfaction amongst heterosexual women without addiction represents a significant hurdle within research. There are several reasons for this: women have different sexual requirements, and their sexual behavior cannot be compared to that of men. Given that this subject area deals largely with 'virgin territory', the focus now turns to general studies of sexual behavior in order to better address the questions posed by this thesis.

Our own study aimed therefore to evaluate patterns of sexual behavior and dysfunction prevalence within buprenorphine and methadone maintenance treatment (Giacomuzzi, 2009). Two questionnaires, in addition to socio-demographic data sets, adapted Relationship Quality Test System (Qualität der Partnerschaftsbeziehung) and EQ-5D (EuroQol), were randomly administered in person by a researcher. A response rate of 100% was obtained. 60 patients (30 buprenorphine; 30 methadone), mean age 30.2 years (IQR 22.5–43.3), were enrolled in the study (Giacomuzzi, 2009).

The study assumed that, in comparison to methadone, the effect of buprenorphine would reduce the additional use of substances. However, this hypothesis could not be established. Neither the substances specified by the various groups in relation to additional use, nor the frequency of consumption were statistically significant.

As a result of this, the study results of Fischer et al. (1999) concerning additional consumption were confirmed. Another assumption of our study was that individuals who take buprenorphine enjoy certain advantages concerning sexual behavior in comparison to those who are administered methadone.

Significant differences were noted between the substitution groups in relation to the question of whether their current sexual life was satisfying. In specific, it is significant that more participants from the buprenorphine group (90%) were satisfied with their current sexual life than participants in the methadone group (63.3%). AT $p = 0.030$, this difference was of considerable statistic significance.

Men on methadone maintenance treatment, but not buprenorphine maintenance treatment, had a high prevalence of sexual excitation disturbances and ability to orgasm in this study.

Significant differences between both groups could be observed regarding sexual excitation disturbances and ability to orgasm. 33.3% of the methadone-maintained group showed significantly higher sexual excitation disturbances ($p = 0.006$) and problems reaching orgasm (40%) ($p = 0.015$) compared with 3.3% respectively 10% within the buprenorphine-maintained group. These results were not affected by sex, since both groups exhibited the same sex distribution (30 men; 30 women).

The study by Bliesener et al. (2004) was confirmed by these results. It should, however, be added that only male participants were represented in the study carried out in 2004. Nevertheless, Bliesener et al. did identify significant results between the methadone and buprenorphine group in relation to libido and virility. In the study presented here, one might assume that these results are influenced by the confounding variable of 'sex', although in light of the identical sex distribution, this was not possible.

	Medication						
	Methadone			Buprenorphine			
	N	Md	IQR	N	Md	IQR	p-value[a]
EQ5D-Index[b]	30	0.752	0.5–0.9	30	0.843	0.7–0.9	0.112
Actual health status in comparison with 12 months ago[c]	30	2.0	1.0–2.0	30	2.0	1.0–2.0	0.725
Self rating regarding acutal health status[d]	30	62.5	43.8–75.0	30	72.5	60.0–80.0	0.032*

[a] * $p < 0.050$; ** $p < 0.001$ (2 sided)
[b] range from -0.3841 to 0.9599 regarding german norm values (the higher the score, the better QOL)
[c] range from 1–3 (1 = better, 2 = equal, 3 = worse)
[d] range from 0–100 (0 = low QOL vs. 100 = high QOL)

Table 1. Quality of Life EQ-5D

A significant correlation between treatment mode and ejaculation praecox, erectile dysfunction, vaginal cramps and sexual aversion could not be observed.
Sexual life satisfaction was scored significantly higher by the buprenorphine-maintained group (90%) compared with the methadone-maintained (63.3%) group (p = 0.030).
The question as to whether climax is experienced during sex was answered with 'mostly' by the median of participants in both substitution groups. The question of how often participants had sex with their partner was answered by participants from the methadone group with a median of 'once a week', and by participants in the buprenorphine group with a median of 'two to three times a week'. However, on average, both groups would like to have sex with their partner 'two to three times a week'. No significant group differences were identified in relation to these three questions concerning sexual behaviour.
In relation to questions concerning the degree of satisfaction with how participants or their partners reacted sexually, consistently high levels of satisfaction (80 to 90%) were recorded. Significant group differences were not identified in relation to these two questions.
Furthermore, sexual partnership was scored significantly higher by women within the buprenorphine-maintained group (p = 0.020).
Further significant differences between the substitution groups were noticed amongst women concerning the question of affection, which was dealt with in the 'Relationship Quality' survey. It was interesting to note that women using methadone as a substitute rated affection higher than women administered the substitute substance Subutex.

		Medication				
		Methadone		Buprenorphine		
		N	[%]	N	[%]	p-value[a]
Is your actual sexual life satisfaying with your partner?	no	11	36.7	3	10.0	
	yes	19	63.3	27	90.0	0.030*
Do you feel comfortable with your sexual reactions?	no	6	20.0	4	13.3	
	yes	24	80.0	26	86.7	0.731
I feel comfortable with my partners sexual reactions.	no	5	16.7	3	10.0	
	yes	25	83.3	27	90.0	0.706

[a] * p < 0.050; ** p < 0.001

Table 2. Sexual satisfaction

Significante differences between the groups were also identified in the area of quality of life. Patients receiving Subutex as a substitute agent gave considerably higher values concerning their self-rated physical health condition than methadone patients.
The self-rated physical health score was significantly higher in the buprenorphine-maintained group compared with the methadone group (p = 0.032). A significant correlation could be found between physical health and substitution mode (p =0.039).

		Substitution substance		
		Methadone	Buprenorphine	
		[%]	[%]	p-value
Is your current sex life with your partner satisfying?	No	36.7	10.0	
	Yes	63.3	90.0	0.030*
I am satisfied with the way in which I react sexually.	No	20.0	13.3	
	Yes	80.0	86.7	0.731
I am satisfied with the way in which my partner reacts sexually.	No	16.7	10.0	
	Yes	83.3	90.0	0.706

* p < 0.050; ** p < 0.001

Table 3. Frequency comparison of sexual satisfaction according to substitution substance

Concerning the self-rated physical health condition on a scale of 0 to 100, participants from the Subutex group achieved a median of 72.5, which was significantly higher than the median value of 62.5 recorded in the methadone group.
In relation to the EQ-5D index, both groups achieved a relatively high index value. The figure for the methadone group was 0.752, whilst the Subutex group even achieved 0.843. Nevertheless, this difference did not reveal any statistical significance. If we consider the answers to 'Current physical health compared with the last 12 months', the median of both groups stated 'Approximately the same'.
In a further step, the connection between the life quality index and the four scales of the relationship survey was calculated. Here, the highest scores on the affection scale amongst men, and the raw scores amongst the female participants, revealed significant results.
In order to verify the results obtained, a covariance test was carried out to explain whether the significant results could be irrefutably attributed to the substitution substance or the intervening covariates. The conclusion of this analysis was that the differences identified were indeed attributable to the different substances.

		Substitution substance		
		Methadone	Buprenorphine	
		[%]	[%]	p-value
Do you masturbate regularly?	No	76.7	60.0	
	Yes	23.3	40.0	0.267
Do you climax (orgasm) when masturbating?	No	30.0	16.7	
	Yes	70.0	83.3	0.360
Do you have arousal disorders?	No	66.7	96.7	
	Yes	33.3	3.3	0.006*
Do you have difficulty reaching orgasm?	No	60.0	90.0	
	Yes	40.0	10.0	0.015*
Do you suffer from premature ejaculation?	No	86.7	100.0	
	Yes	13.3	0.0	0.483
Do you suffer from erectile dysfunction?	No	93.3	100.0	
	Yes	6.7	0.0	1.000
Do you have vaginal cramps during sex?	No	93.3	100.0	
	Yes	6.7	0.0	1.000
Do you have cramp-like pain during sex?	No	93.3	100.0	
	Yes	6.7	0.0	1.000
Do you have sexual aversion?	No	73.3	93.3	
	Yes	26.7	6.7	0.330

* $p < 0.050$; ** $p < 0.001$

Table 4. Frequency comparison concerning questions on sexuality according to substitution substance

4. Conclusions

Substitution therapy has become the main form of post-acute treatment of opiate addicts. Despite this, the most suitable substitution substance remains a topic of controversial debate today. Alongside methadone, which is by far the most researched substance, buprenorphine is now increasingly used.

On the one hand, methadone substitution has become established as suitable treatment worldwide, given that it not only has a stabilising and health-maintaining effect, but also leads to an improvement in social rehabilitation (Giacomuzzi, 2009). A central argument put forward by those in favour of methadone against buprenorphine is the danger of intravenous consumption of this substance, through which the 'rush' is achieved, which is missing with oral administration. In contrast, methadone opposers contend that precisely the low euphoric effect of methadone causes problems with the acceptance of the substitute and leads to increased parallel consumption behavior.

On the other hand, in light of the diverse side effects of methadone, new substances like buprenorphine are becoming increasingly popular. Proponents affirm that when compared

directly with methadone, buprenorphine presents more advantages. A wide range of studies have shown that even in high doses, buprenorphine causes fewer side effects than methadone, presents a lower dependence potential, increases drive and has anti-depressive properties.
The standard substitution therapy continues to be methadone. All new drugs or substances used must be able to compete with the success or failure experiences of traditional methadone substitution (Giacomuzzi, 2009).
The clarification of the individual needs of different groups of drug addicts seems particularly important for the future (Giacomuzzi, 2009). Therapy studies have proven that psychosocial measures, coupled with substitution, achieve significantly better effects than psychopharmacotherapy alone. The current offer of drug clinics, private associations, etc. is not sufficient to meet patients' needs.
Opioid maintenance treatment, primarily methadone, appears to be associated with alteration of serum levels of hormones related to normal sexual function.
In males, opioids may act via: (1) interference with the normal production of hypothalamic and pituitary regulatory hormones, (2) elevation of serum prolactin, (3) direct action on the testes to suppress testosterone production (Brown & Zueldorff, 2007).
While elimination of other common medical and psychiatric etiologies for sexual dysfunction is warranted, replacement of abnormally low serum testosterone may effectively treat libido or erectile dysfunction, and potentially delayed orgasm or anorgasmia. Replacement of abnormally low androgens in women on opioid maintenance treatment may also improve libido as well as mood.
Abnormalities in the menstrual cycle are thought to be transient and may not require alteration of opioid maintenance treatment dosing. Patients with refractory sexual dysfunction and a stable course in terms of their opioid use disorder may correspond to reduction in the dose of their opioid maintenance treatment agent, with methadone likely being of greater significance here than buprenorphine (Brown & Zueldorff, 2007).
Sexual behavior is not only of basic biological importance, but also of central social importance. Not only does it perpetuate the human species, but it is the central behavior around which families are formed and defined, a vital aspect of the psychological well-being of individuals, and a component of a variety of social problems.
There has been very little research on ED among buprenorphine patients. Men on methadone maintenance treatment, but not buprenorphine maintenance treatment, had a high prevalence of sexual excitation disturbances and ability to orgasm. Orgasm dysfunction seems to be a special case and may respond to methadone dose (Giacomuzzi, 2009).
In light of the paucity of studies in the area of sexual dysfunction as an adverse effect of buprenorphine, more research is needed, utilizing larger patient populations and examining more thoroughly specific types of dysfunction in both male and female populations.
Future studies of sexual dysfunction in opioid-treated persons should examine the potential benefits of dose reduction, androgen replacement, and choice of opioid (Giacomuzzi, 2009).
Practitioners should screen for sexual dysfunction in men receiving opioid replacement treatment. Orgasm dysfunction seems to be a special case and may correspond more to methadone dose. Future studies of sexual dysfunction in opioidtreated persons should examine the potential benefits of dose reduction, androgen replacement, and choice of opioid (Giacomuzzi, 2009).
Therapy and patient care should be structured in a more flexible manner.

5. References

Bliesener, N., Albrecht, S., Schwager, A., Weckbecker, K., Lichtermann, D. and Klingmuller, D. (2005): Plasma testosterone and sexual function in men receiving buprenorphine maintenance for opioid dependence. *J. Clin. Endocrinol. Metab.* Vol. 90, pp. 203-206.

Brown, R.T. & Zueldorff, M. (2007). Opioid Substitution with Methadone and Buprenorphine: Sexual Dysfunction as a Side Effect of Therapy. Heroin Addiction and Related Clinical Problems. Vol. 9(1), pp. 35-44

Büsing, S., Hoppe, C. & Liedtke, R. (2001). Sexuelle Zufriedenheit von Frauen – Entwicklung und Ergebnisse eines Fragebogens. PPmP Psychother Psychosom med Psychol 2001, Vol. 51, pp. 68–75.

Fischer, G., Gombas, W., Eder, H., Jagsch, R., Peternell, A., Stühlinger, G., Pezawas, L., Aschauer, H.N. & Kasper, S. (1999). Buprenorphin versus methadone maintenance for the treatment of opioid dependence. *Addiction*, Vol. 94(9), pp. 1337–1347.

Giacomuzzi S.M., Garber, K. & Riemer, Y. (2011). Patient-specific perceptions and effects on Sublingual Suboxone® maintenance treatment and their impact regarding the acceptance as treatment choice – a semi-qualitative analysis. *Gobal Addiction Conference Lissabon*. to be published

Giacomuzzi, S.M., Khreis, A, Riemer, A., Garber, K. & Ertl, M. (2009). Buprenorphine and Methadone Maintenance Treatment – Sexual Behaviour and Dysfunction Prevalence. *Letters in Drug Design & Discovery*, 2009, Vol. 6, pp. 13

Giacomuzzi, S. (2008). A Contribution to the Understanding of the Addiction Phenomenon, IUP, Innsbruck University Press, ISBN 13: 978-3-902571-28-1, Innsbruck, Austria

Giacomuzzi, S.M., Ertl, M., Riemer, Y., Kemmler, G., Rössler, H., Hinterhuber, H. & Kurz, M. (2005). Sublingual buprenorphine and methadone maintenance treatment - a 3 year follow up of quality of life assessment. *The Scientific World Journal*, Vol.5, pp. 452-468

Giacomuzzi, S.M.; Riemer, Y.; Ertl, M.; Kemmler, G.; Rössler, H.; Hinterhuber, H. & Kurz, M. (2003). Buprenorphine versus methadone maintenance treatment in an ambulant setting - a health-related quality of life assessment. *Addiction*, Vol.98, pp. 693-702.

Haebere, E.J. (1981, 1983). The Sex Atlas. New popular Reference Edition Revised and Expanded. 1983, The Continuum Publishing Company, 575 Lexington Avenue, New York, N.Y. 10022

Mattick R.P., Kimber, J., Breen, C. & Davoli, M. (2004). Buprenorphine maintenance versus placebo or methadone maintenance for opioid dependence. Cochrane Database of Systematic Reviews (Online), Vol. 3, CD002207

Mendelson, J. H., Inturrisi, C. E., Renault, P. & Senay, E. C. (1976): Effects of acetylmethadol on plasma testosterone. *Clin. Pharmacol. Ther.* 19, pp. 371-374.

Mendelson, J. H. & Mello, N. K. (1975). Plasma testosterone levels during chronic heroin use and protracted astinence. A study of Hong Kong addicts. *Clin. Pharmacol. Ther.* 17, pp. 529-533.

Mendelson, J. H., Meyer, R. E., Ellingboe, J., Mirin, S. M. & McDougle, M. (1975). Effects of heroin and methadone on plasma cortisol and testosterone. *J. Pharmacol. Exp. Ther.* 195, pp. 296-302.

Petry, N.M., Bickel, W.K. & Badger, G.J. (2001). Examining the limits of the buprenorphine interdosing interval: daily, every-third-day and every-fifth-day dosing regimens, *Addiction*, Vol. 96, pp. 823-834

Teusch, L., Scherbaum, N., Bohme, H., Bender, S., Eschmann-Mehl, G. and Gastpar, M. (1995). Different patterns of sexual dysfunctions associated with psychiatric disorders and psychopharmacological treatment. Results of an investigation by semistructured interview of schizophrenic and neurotic patients and methadone-substituted opiate addicts. *Pharmacopsychiatry*, Vol. 28, pp. 84-92

Quaglio, G., Lugoboni, F., Pattaro, C., Melara, B., Mezzelani, P. & Jarlais D.C. (2008). Erectile dysfunction in male heroin users, receiving methadone and buprenorphine maintenance treatment. *Drug and Alcohol Dependence*, Vol. 94, p.p 12–18

3

Sexual Dysfunction Among Cancer Survivors

Atara Ntekim
Department of Radiation Oncology, College of Medicine, University of Ibadan
Nigeria

1. Introduction

"Sexual and reproductive health and wellbeing are essential if people are to have responsible, safe and satisfying sexual lives. Sexual health requires a positive approach to human sexuality and an understanding of the complex factors that shape human sexual behaviour. These factors affect whether the expression of sexuality leads to sexual health and well- being or to sexual behaviour that put people at risk or make them vulnerable to sexual and reproductive ill- health. Health program managers, policy - makers and care providers need to understand and promote the potentially positive role sexuality can play in peoples' lives and to build health services that can promote sexually health societies." - (WHO 2006)

There is increasing number of cancer survivors worldwide. A lot of them experience sexual dysfunction for a long time which can last beyond ten years post treatment. Sexual dysfunction can occur as a result of any aspect of cancer and cancer treatment. Sexual functioning and/or satisfaction have been found to be of concern to many cancer survivors. Sexual function can be affected by physical or emotional trauma especially if the genitals are affected and can adversely affect the quality of life of the patients. Sexual dysfunction includes erectile dysfunction in males and disruption in the sexual response cycle (sexual desire, excitement, arousal, orgasm and resolution) and dyspareunia in women. There are differences in the pattern of sexual dysfunction between males and females as females may be able to cope better than males emotionally. Bonini-Colmano et al. (2007) noted that malignant diseases have a strong influence in quality of life, sexuality being one of the most affected variables. In their study to determine the prevalence of sexual dysfunction in a cohort of patients with cancer and its relationship with the following: pain, fatigue, nausea, vomiting, mechanisms of adaptation to stress, anxiety and depression, questionnaires were used which included treatment, adverse events, Zimong and Snaith depression and anxiety scale, sexual dysfunction questionnaire, coping strategies of Tobin David, Hopwood body image scale and the analogical visual test for pain evaluation. Sixty four patients were evaluated. Seventy two percent were women and median age was 50 years. Libido was absent in 50%; this was associated with gender (better in men; p=0,05) and the presence of pain (p=0,05) and fatigue (p=0,05) but not with age. All patients who had intact libido also had arousal and orgasms; this was more prevalent in men than in women and in subjects younger than 60 years. Arousal was absent in 47% of cases. Forty four percent of men had erectile dysfunction; this was present in all patients older than 60 years. Frequency of intercourses was decreased in 75%. Fifty eight percent of patients said that their sexuality was better before the diagnosis of their disease. Interestingly, 85% didn't talk to their doctors about their sexual problems. The study concluded that one out of 2 patients had sexual dysfunction, predominantly women and that sexuality was affected mainly by pain and fatigue. Although normal libido was present in all ages, subjects older than 60 years had less arousal and orgasms.

The age of the patients also determines the extent of the problem. Testicular cancer for example is more common among youths. At this age group, the patients are either about to get married or in early stage of their family life. Sexual problem at this stage can be grievous and very traumatizing. Prostate cancer on the other hand is common among the elderly who would have completed their family and may be more concerned about survival than sexual activities. Sexual issues may therefore not be of prominence among this age group. The site of the disease also determines the extent of the problem. A male patient with cancer of the penis treated with amputation of the penis will experience more sexual dysfunction than a patient with testicular cancer who has a testicle removed. In females, a breast cancer patient who had the affected breast removed (mastectomy) will experience more sexuality issues than a female counterpart who had only the lump removed (lumpectomy). (Ofman 1995) Likewise, a female patient treated for cervical cancer with radiotherapy will experience more sexual problems than a female patient treated for head and neck cancer with radiotherapy.

Survivors of cancer of various anatomical sites experience various degrees of sexual dysfunction. After treatment, approximately 20% to 30% of breast cancer survivors, 80% of prostate cancer survivors, 37% of Hodgkin's survivors, and 58% of head and neck cancer survivors report sexual difficulties. (Elyse et al., 2009) Changes in body image, pain, and loss of desire result from both cancer and its treatment; long-term physical and psychological side effects from cancer treatments can affect sexual functioning. Long-term psychological responses, such as depression and anxiety about cancer, may alter the survivor's ability for intimacy and sexuality.

Sexual dysfunction therefore is an important issue that affects many cancer survivors who are increasingly being cared for by health personnel. It is noted that sexual dysfunction among these group of patients is never addressed by most of their care givers during follow up management. Many effective behavioural and pharmacological treatments for sexual dysfunction exist. However, to identify cancer survivors who may benefit from these treatments, conversations about sexual dysfunctions must be initiated. Survivors express a desire to be able to discuss sexual issues with medical professionals. However, there are barriers to these conversations for both patients and physicians. A public opinion poll of 500 adults in the United States showed that 85% would be willing to talk to their physicians if they had a sexual problem. However, 71% did not think that their physicians would be responsive or helpful, and 68% were concerned that their physicians would be uncomfortable and also reports from some studies found that lack of knowledge, expertise, time, and comfort are barriers to these conversations. (Bober et al., 2009)

2. Aim

The aim of this chapter is to highlight sexual health issues among cancer survivors so that clinicians and care givers can be able to predict this sequel and incorporate measures as early as possible towards prevention, reduction, assessment using appropriate instruments and management of this important condition among patients thereby improving the sexuality aspect of their quality of life.

3. Methods

Available literature (hard and electronic copies) including the authors work relevant to this topic were consulted and evaluated. The sexuality component of the authors work on quality of life of head and neck cancer patients seen at The Radiotherapy Department, University College Hospital, Ibadan Nigeria (yet to be published) is reported .

4. Findings and discussion

The findings together with relevant discussion pertaining to common group of malignancies are as follows:

4.1 Female breast cancer survivors

Breast cancer is a common cancer among women and survival has increased over time especially if treatment is commenced early. Five year survival has reached about 97% especially in the developed countries with early disease. (Thors et al., 2001) This implies that a lot of women will live long and are likely to experience sexual dysfunction. With breast cancer the term "survivors" is used here to refer to women who have completed surgery, chemotherapy/hormonal and/or radiation therapy for the treatment of breast cancer. Most breast cancer survivors experience about 15% reduction in sexual satisfaction after treatment (Bukovic et al., 2005). Approximately 20-30% of breast cancer survivors experience sexual problems including general sexual disruption, decreased frequency of intercourse, and difficulties reaching orgasm that may persist 20 years post-treatment (Alfano et al., 2007).The reported prevalence of this problem varies greatly, partly due to the various methods and instruments used in their assessment. In terms of specific sexual difficulties, the most common current symptoms reported in this study were absence of sexual desire (48%), reduced sexual desire (64%), anorgasmia (44%), lubrication difficulties (42%), and dyspareunia (38%) while two or more problems were present in about 97% of the participants. These findings show that certain problems appear to be related to the desire stage of sexual activity (e.g. loss of interest in sex), while others appear to be related to the arousal stage (e.g. lubrication difficulties) and the orgasmic stage (e.g. anorgasmy).

In a study among sexually active and recurrence free breast cancer patients who had completed surgery, chemotherapy, and radiation therapy, 64% of the women reported an absence of sexual desire, 38% suffered from dyspareunia, and 42% experienced lubrication problems Vaginismus, brief intercourse and female orgasmic disorder were reported by 30% of the subjects. Thirty-six percent suffered from sexual dysfunction before treatment, which worsened in about 27%, while in 49% of women sexual problems arose mainly after chemotherapy (26%) or surgery (12%). About one-half experienced changes in the relationship with their partner (Barni and Mondin 1997). In another study of breast cancer survivors, sexual dysfunction occurred more frequently in women who had received chemotherapy and in younger women who were no longer menstruating and depression was an important determinant of lower sexual desire, and survivors on antidepressants had greater problems with arousal and achieving orgasm. (Melisko et al., 2010) In a retrospective study of breast cancer among young females in Nigeria aged 40 years and

below earlier reported by the author, 46 % of the patients reported loss of libido (Ntekim et al., 2009). Another study revealed that women diagnosed at age ≤ 40 years had significant less sexual interest after treatment than women over 40 years (Morrow, 2011).
Survivors with upper extremity lymphedema following breast cancer treatment also experience sexual dysfunction with upper extremity lymphedema as an additional predisposing factor. Sixty-nine women presenting for rehabilitation treatment for upper extremity lymphedema (UEL) were assessed by physical examination and validated self-report assessment instruments measuring demographics, psychological distress, sexual functioning, social support, coping style, pain and functional status by Passik and colleagues (2007). Their analyses revealed that women with UEL had high levels of psychological distress, and high levels of sexual, functional and social dysfunction. There were no linear relationships between severity of UEL and levels of distress. Women with UEL in their dominant hand, however, had more distress and less overall sexual satisfaction than those with UEL in their non-dominant limb. Women with pain of any intensity were the most distressed, and had the most significant difficulties in psychological and physical functioning. Women with pain also perceived significantly less interpersonal support than those without pain. Virtually none were receiving pain treatment. An avoidant coping style and low perceived social support were significant correlates of psychological distress. The study concluded that UEL poses significant functional, social and sexual functioning problems in women following breast cancer treatment and that these patients may also benefit from psychological support and sexual therapy in addition to physical rehabilitation.
There are therefore multiple predisposing factors for sexual dysfunction including pre-existing sexual problems, negative sexual self-schemas, (cognitive generalizations regarding sexual aspects of the self; they represent a core component of one's sexuality) and normal age-related changes in sexual functioning. Physical consequences of treatment like absence of one breast, scar on the breast and upper extremity lymphedema are also important predisposing factors. Partners sexual problems and psychological reaction to the diagnosis of cancer are also contributory. Physiologic changes induced by chemotherapy are also important contributors. Induction of premature menopause can result in an estrogen deficiency state that increases the likelihood of hot flashes and poor vaginal lubrication that may contribute to sexual dysfunction (Kaplan, 1991)

4.1.1 Sexual dysfunction and chemotherapy

Compared to breast cancer women who were not treated with adjuvant chemotherapy, women treated with adjuvant chemotherapy are 5.7 times more likely to report vaginal dryness, 3 times more likely to report decreased libido, 5.5 times more likely to report dyspareunia, and 7.1 times more likely to report difficulty reaching orgasm.(Ganze etal., 1998). Chemotherapy therefore affects sexual functioning in women though the extent may vary according to different drug regimen and patients age.

4.1.2 Sexual dysfunction and hormonal therapy

It has been found that the incidence of vaginal dryness, dyspareunia, and loss of sexual interest in women taking Aromatase Inhibitors (AIs) was significant. These symptoms were particularly bothersome in women who experienced acute chemotherapy induced menopause as reported by Fallowfield et al., 2004. In the 5 year follow up in this study, vaginal discharge was less frequently bothersome with anastrozole than Tamoxifen (1.2%

vs. 5.2%) but vaginal dryness (18.5% vs. 9.1%), dyspareunia (17.3% vs. 8.1%), and reduced libido (34.0% vs. 26.1%) were all more common with anastrozole compared with Tamoxifen (Cella 2006). In the quality of life sub-study for the Intergroup Exemestane Study (IES), loss of libido was common and did not differ between groups receiving Tamoxifen for 5 years compared to those patients who switched over to exemestane after 2-3 years of Tamoxifen. There were no differences between the Tamoxifen or exemestane groups for vaginal dryness, discomfort with intercourse, and vaginal irritation (Fallowfield 2006).Even in patients without a diagnosis of breast cancer, hormonal therapies appear to have an impact on sexual function. Analysis of quality of life data from the Study of Raloxifene and Tamoxifen (STAR) prevention trial found that a higher percentage of women randomized to the Tamoxifen arm remained sexually active compared to women in the Raloxifene arm. Among sexually active participants, women randomized to the Raloxifene group experienced significantly more dyspareunia, greater difficulties with sexual interest, sexual arousal, and sexual enjoyment, but no significant difference in the ability to experience an orgasm (Land 2006).

Ganz et al (1999) , found that among women 1 to 5 years post treatment, sexual problems (as measured by the CARES and the Watts Sexual Functioning Scale) were more common in women who had received chemotherapy. Lindley et al. (1998 as cited in Thors 2001), reported an interaction between age and chemotherapy in that the greatest negative change in sexual functioning (as measured by a series of questions that included items measuring sexual satisfaction and interest) occurred in premenopausal women who experienced chemotherapy-induced amenorrhea. Under oestrogen deprivation, with time, the mucosal and stromal tissues of the vagina, urethra, and trigone of the bladder undergo atrophy, resulting in decreased tissue elasticity and fluid secretion. This may lead to symptomatic vaginal dryness and irritation as well as dyspareunia. Oestrogen deprivation also leads to an elevation in vaginal pH which may increase the risk of vaginal and urinary tract infections.

4.1.3 Interventions

Study Instruments:

A number of study instruments have been used in sexual dysfunction studies in breast cancer survivors. The two more commonly used ones are Sexual History Form and the sexual summary subscale of the Cancer Rehabilitation Evaluation System (CARES). The Sexual History Form was developed by Schover and Jensen (1988, cited in Thors et al., 2001) and is composed of 27 multiple choice questions assessing sexual functioning, frequency, and satisfaction with sexual activity. This questionnaire has been standardized and norms from a healthy community sample are available for comparison purposes. The CARES is a quality-of-life instrument that includes an 8-item subscale measuring sexual interest and sexual dysfunction. The CARES has been shown to have adequate reliability and validity, and normative scores are available for cancer patients (Thors et al., 2001).

Other study questionnaires include Watts Sexual Functioning Questionnaire (442-13, sexual dysfunction subscale of The European Organization for Research and Treatment of Cancer [EORTC] QLQ-C30), Derogatis Sexual Functioning Inventory (DSFI), Arizona Sexual Experience Scale (ASEX) and Female Sexual Functioning Index (FSFI). Revised Dyadic Adjustment Scale can be used to assess partner relationship variables so also with Marital Satisfaction Inventory-Revised (MAI-R) (Stead 2003).

Communication with women concerning sexual life is vital. Psychotherapy and behavioural approaches has been shown to be useful in managing these patients. Pharmacologic agents especially non estrogenic topical agents for specific problems like vaginal dryness are recommended. However a thorough assessment to determine which aspect of sexual function is affected can help in prescribing suitable approach to management. This can be done using more detailed study instruments. The commencement of pelvic floor muscle exercises, use of vaginal moisturizer to alleviate vaginal dryness and olive oil as lubricant during intercourse has been shown to improve sexual function in breast cancer survivors. (Juraskova 2011)

4.2 Genito-urinary cancer survivors

Survivors of cancer of the genito-urinary system do experience sexual dysfunction of which some are peculiar to affected organs. Some organs like the urinary bladder are closely related to sex organs and can directly affect sexual functions during the course of the disease and treatment. Post treatment effects like ovarian failure after chemotherapy and pelvic radiotherapy in females can have effects on sexual functions of survivors.

4.2.1 Testicular cancer

Testicular cancer is the most common cancer of young men in their 20s and 30s. Since the advent of effective multiagent cisplatinum-based chemotherapy, the majority of patients are cured. This disease occurs during the peak period of reproductive life and at a key time for career and family. As cured testicular patients have a long life expectancy, sexual function becomes an important issue. It has been found that hormonal dysfunction is frequent after the diagnosis of testicular cancer and treatment can have an additional detrimental effect. This can have a significant impact on the sexual life of the survivor and contribute to other health problems. Most patients, however, remain fertile though this can be affected by their treatment. Long-lasting sexual problems after therapy for testicular cancer are present in approximately one-fifth of patients undergoing treatment for testicular germ cell tumour. On the other hand, the majority of patients have not reported infertility or sexual dysfunction-related symptoms (Hartmann et al., 1999). In a study by Huddart and colleagues, the testicular module of the EORTC QLQ C-30 Questionnaire, which consists of six questions directed at sexual function and sexual satisfaction and two additional questions about masculinity and concerns about fathering children, was used. Overall sexual function from the analysis seemed to be satisfactory with 83% of patients expressing satisfaction in their sexual relationships with their partner with no differences between treatment groups. Compared to surveillance there was a tendency for treated groups to have less sexual activity and less interest in sex. This was only statistically significant for patients treated with chemotherapy and radiotherapy (CRT) and less interest in sex was of borderline significance for CRT and radiotherapy (RT). Additionally, radiotherapy treatment was associated with reduced sexual enjoyment compared with patients on surveillance (Huddart et al., 2005) The Derogatis Interview for Sexual Functioning-II Self-Report-Male questionnaire can also be used to assess sexual dysfunction in males (Greenfield et al.,2010).

4.2.2 Prostate cancer

Erectile dysfunction is common after prostatectomy because of the interference with the nerves. The extent being different with different methods of surgery as some have more nerve sparing effects than others.

In comparison with prostatectomy, patients treated with external beam radiation report less long-lasting urinary symptoms, but more bowel side effects, with no difference in global quality of life. Sexual disorders are initially less important with external beam radiation but increase over time. Brachytherapy shows no sexual function preservation benefit relative to external beam radiation and may be less favourable with more urinary sequelae. The association of hormonal therapy and external beam radiation decreases the quality of life of the patients, with a negative impact on vitality, sexuality and increase urinary disorders. Intensity-modulated radiotherapy (IMRT) seems to better preserve the long-term digestive quality of life in comparison with conformal radiation therapy (Joly et al., 2010).
Radical surgical prostatectomy for cancer is performed by the perineal, retropubic, or transpubic routes. Surveys of patients undergoing either retropubic or perineal prostatectomy have reported comparable findings, with estimates of diminished erectile capabilities or complete erectile failure after surgery for 90% of the patients. The incidence of ejaculation difficulties with or without concomitant erectile failure is estimated as occurring for 78% of the retropubic and 100% of the perineal prostatectomy patients. If hormone therapy and/or orchiectomy are additionally used after either surgical procedure, virtually 100% of the patients experience erectile failure and ejaculation difficulties. These estimates are three to four times higher than those for patients treated for benign conditions with less extensive surgery (Andersen 1985). The sexual domain of the Expanded Prostate Cancer Index (EPIC) questionnaire can be used to assess prostate cancer survivors.

4.2.3 Bladder cancer

Early bladder cancer is treated by transurethral resection and there may be minimal sexual dysfunction. Cystectomy is associated with reduction in desire and erectile function in about 30% of male patients while sexual excitement and orgasm is impaired in women. (Anderson 1985) A comprehensive, disease specific measure of health related quality of life in patients with localised bladder cancer has been developed by Gilbert et al., (2010).

4.3 Gynaecological cancer survivors

Modalities of treatment comprising of surgery, chemotherapy, radiotherapy and hormonal therapy either single or in various combinations are used to treat gynaecological malignancies. All these modes have the potential to affect sexual functions of the patients. Gynaecological malignancies have the ability to affects a woman's sexual wellbeing primarily as the sexual reproductive organs are involved. Altered sexual functioning is the most affected aspect of quality of life of gynaecological cancer survivors occurring in 40-100% of patients compared to 19%-50% of the healthy outpatient population (Andersen, 1985).

4.3.1 Cervical cancer

The two modes of treatment for early disease, radical hysterectomy and radiation therapy, are equally common for early stage cervical cancer. Surgical treatment allows ovarian preservation for premenopausal women, but does cause vaginal shortening, which has contributed to coital discomfort (Andersen & Hacker 1983). Radiation therapy destroys ovarian functioning and causes vaginal atrophy and stenosis. Dyspareunia from lack of lubrication, tenderness of the vagina, and post coital bleeding have been resultant problems. Comparable outcome with 29% and 33% of radiation and hysterectomy patients, respectively, reporting subsequent sexual difficulties have been reported (Andersen 1985).

Some studies demonstrated that women with early stage cervical cancer receiving hysterectomy and radiotherapy suffered a number of short-term sexual difficulties such as dyspareunia, problems during intercourse and lack of sexual satisfaction, but that by 6 months after the surgery these problems had often reduced. However, some sexual difficulties persisted, in particular lack of sexual interest and lack of lubrication. In contrast, women with advanced, recurrent, or persistent cervical cancer experienced prolonged problems with vaginal lubrication, lack of orgasm, and lower frequency of intercourse, in addition to reduced sexual interest, throughout the 24 months post diagnosis (Stead 2004)
The Female Sexual Function Index (FSFI) questionnaire and ALARM model are useful questionnaires to assess sexual function in these patients (Andersen 1990).
In a study by Lindau ST et al.(2007)sexual problems were significantly more prevalent among very long term (>25 years) survivors of cervical and vaginal cancers than in population-based comparison group. For example, the prevalence of dyspareunia (pain during intercourse) and difficulty lubricating were, respectively, nearly 7 and 3 times higher among survivors. Survivors were also significantly more likely than those in the population-based sample to exhibit complex sexual morbidity, defined as concurrent sexual problems in three or more of seven domains , and to report avoiding sex because of sexual problems (62% versus 43%). In the same study, 62% of survivors reported that a doctor had never initiated a conversation about the effects of cancer or treatments for genital tract cancer on sexuality and Bivariate analysis revealed that a conversation with a physician about the sexual effects of genital tract cancer and cancer treatment is associated with significantly fewer sex morbidities. Some studies show that education on vaginal lubricants, moisturizers, and dilator use (as needed) can decrease the morbidity of vaginal atrophy (Carter et al., 2011).

4.3.2 Vulval cancer

Surgical treatment is commonly used for treating vulval carcinoma. This has some effects on sexual performance of the patients and various patterns of sexual dysfunction have been reported. A survey of 18 patients treated with wide local excision rather than vulvectomy for microinvasive disease indicated that all women continued to be orgasmic during sexual activity, in contrast to two radical vulvectomy patients who reported loss of orgasmic ability and dyspareunia. (Andersen 1985) A retrospective study of women who received radical surgery indicated discrepancies between the actual and the preferred frequency of sexual activities such as intercourse and a limited capacity for sexual arousal among these patients. Interestingly, orgasmic responsiveness is reported by women who had and who had not undergone clitoral excision at the time of vulvectomy (Thuesen et al., 1992). Another study has shown that more than half of women with vulval cancer experience sexual problems, with those women undergoing local vulval excision for vulval dysplasia experiencing the most problems. While these, in part, are related to anatomic changes, inadequate counselling and poor advice were contributing factors. A small study described how vulvectomy was associated with altered body image and arousal difficulties, and suggested that risk factors for sexual problems were age, depression, poor performance status, and preoperative sexual dysfunction. These findings demonstrate the need for appropriate counselling and advice for women with vulval cancer. (Green et al., 2000)

4.3.3 Endometrial cancer

Women with endometrial cancer are usually older and postmenopausal and their treatment often involves surgery plus radiotherapy and so surgery and radiation induced vaginal difficulties can occur. The pattern of sexual difficulties may be similar to those with cervical cancer of similar age group.

4.3.4 Ovarian cancer

Ovarian cancer is usually treated with a hysterectomy (including oophorectomy), and chemotherapy. Few of them also have adjuvant radiotherapy. These can all affect sexual functioning, through a decrease in oestrogen production resulting in vaginal atrophy and dryness. There can be hot flushes and loss of sexual interest resulting from changes in body and hormonal levels especially if the patients were pre menopausal prior to treatment. A study of 200 survivors of ovarian cancer showed that over 50% reported worsened sexual function (Stewart et al., 2001)

A cross-sectional study in 232 women with ovarian cancer showed that ovarian cancer is also associated with low sexual desire (47% reported no/little desire), vaginal dryness (experienced in 80% of women having sexual intercourse in the last month), dyspareunia (in 62%), and problems with orgasm (in 75%). This study also evaluated predictors of sexual activity and found that being married, being under 56 years, not receiving treatment, good self-esteem/body image, and length of time since end of treatment were all associated with being sexually active. This paper compared the findings of the research with studies in breast cancer and healthy postmenopausal women and concluded that although low desire, vaginal dryness, and dyspareunia occur in these other groups; the problems are more common and more severe in women with ovarian cancer. (Stead, 2004). A study of survivors of ovarian cancer found that about 80% of them who were sexually active before treatment reported vaginal dryness. This can lead to dyspareunia and subsequent fear of possible pain during vaginal penetration may contribute to the loss of interest in sex. (Carmack-Taylor et al., 2004).

EORTIC QLQ OV 28 is a useful questionnaire in assessing sexual dysfunction among ovarian cancer survivors.

The possible sexual problems caused by cancer treatment in females are presented in table 1 below.

Treatment	Low Sexual Desire	Less Vaginal Moisture	Reduced Vaginal Size	Painful Intercourse	Trouble Reaching Orgasm	Infertility
Chemotherapy	Sometimes	Often	Sometimes	Often	Rarely	Often
Pelvic radiation therapy	Rarely	Often	Often	Often	Rarely	Often
Radical hysterectomy	Rarely	Often[b]	Often	Rarely	Rarely	Always
Radical cystectomy	Rarely	Often[b]	Always	Sometimes	Rarely	Always
Abdominoperineal (A-P) resection	Rarely	Often[b]	Sometimes	Sometimes	Rarely	Sometimes[b]
Total pelvic exenteration with vaginal reconstruction	Sometimes	Always	Sometimes	Sometimes	Sometimes	Always
Radical vulvectomy	Rarely	Never	Sometimes	Often	Sometimes	Never
Conization of the cervix	Never	Never	Never	Rarely	Never	Rarely
Oophorectomy (removal of one tube and ovary)	Rarely	Never[b]	Never[b]	Rarely	Never	Rarely
Oophorectomy (removal of both tubes and ovaries)	Rarely	Often[b]	Sometimes[b]	Sometimes[b]	Rarely	Always
Mastectomy or radiation to the breast	Rarely	Never	Never	Never	Rarely	Never
Tamoxifen therapy for breast or uterine cancer	Sometimes	Often	Sometimes	Sometimes	Rarely	Always
Androgen therapy	Never	Never	Never	Never	Never	Uncertain

b Vaginal dryness and size changes should not occur if one ovary is retained or if hormone therapy is given.

Table 1. Female sexual problems caused by cancer treatment. (Adapted from American Cancer Society Inc. 2009 as cited in Audette and Waterman 2010).

4.4 Gastro intestinal cancer survivors

Survivors of gastrointestinal malignancies also experience sexual disorders. Although studies in most sites are not easily available, few reports show that survivors of these cancer site also experience sexual dysfunction.

4.4.1 Colorectal cancer survivors

Colorectal cancer is quite common all over the world including Europe and America. Surgical resection is an effective treatment modality for early diseases. The surgical approach differs according to the location of the tumour. Low lying tumours are located 0-5 cm from the anal verge and abdomino- perineal resection is the approach commonly used resulting in permanent colostomy. A review by Sprangers et al. (2003) noted that this operation disrupts nerve fibres associated with sexual function more in men than in women. It also noted that low or high anterior resection used in the treatment of tumours located more than 5cm from the anal verge (lower or upper colon) which are sphincter sparing, also disrupts some nerves associated with sexual function especially if ultra low anastomosis are used. In a study on survivors after chemo-radiotherapy for rectal cancer using EORTIC QLQ-CR38, The scores for "sexual functioning" and "enjoyment" were low. Men had more sexual problems than females (62.5 vs. 25 mean scores respectively). (Tiv et al, .2010). Erectile dysfunction was also reported among men and the presence of colostomy was reported to further reduce sexual functioning in males but not in females.

Several retrospective studies of sexual functioning after excision of the rectum for cancer have been conducted. For men, estimates of sexual dysfunctions have ranged from 32% to 59% for sexual desire, from 28% to 76% for erectile difficulties and from 66% to 86% for ejaculation disruption (Andersen, 1985). Estimates for women from one investigation reported that 28% of the sample had reduced desire and 21 % reported genital numbness or dyspareunia. (Kuchenhoff 1981 as cited in Andersen 1985)

Laparoscopic surgical techniques have been used in resection of colorectal cancers with reported equivalence in tumour clearance with conventional open techniques. It has additional advantage of less pain, reduced hospital stay and earlier return to normal function. In a retrospective assessment for rectal dysfunction in colorectal cancer patients who had laparoscopic resection, Aquah et al. (2002) reported that a significant difference in sexual function in males but not females was noted. Seven of the 15 sexually active men in the laparoscopic group reported impotence or impaired ejaculation while only one of the 22 patients in the open surgery group had such complain. (P=0.004). The study concluded that laparoscopic resection of colorectal cancer was associated with more sexual dysfunction than open surgical resection.

4.4.2 Hepatocellular cancer (HCC)

Patients with hepatocellular carcinoma also experience sexual dysfunction. In a study by Steel et al., (2005) comparing sexual dysfunction among hepatocellular cancer patients and chronic liver disease (CLD) patients, reported that with regards to the differences between HCC patients and those with CLD with respect to sexual problems, the rates of sexual morbidity were found to be higher in patients diagnosed with HCC for the majority of the sexual problems, including hypoactive sexual desire disorder (26% vs. 18%), sexual aversion disorder (18% vs. 5%), male orgasmic disorder (13% vs. 5%), premature ejaculation (17% vs. 5%), and dyspareunia (12% vs. 5%). The only disorder in which CLD patients reported a higher prevalence than HCC patients was male erectile disorder (21% vs. 17%) Male patients had more sexual problems than the general population. The study also noted that co morbid conditions like hypertension, diabetes mellitus and cardio vascular diseases were more prevalent among HCC patients and medications for these conditions could add to their sexual problems.

4.4.3 Anal cancer

Majority of patients treated for anal cancer experience sexual dysfunction. A study using split course chemo radiotherapy for the treatment of anal cancer among 58 patients reported that fifty percent of patients maintained an interest in having sexual relations but 100% of male patients had difficulty maintaining an erection. Forty-four percent of men qualified the erectile dysfunction as severe (# 4 on the scale: very much). Among women, 65% had no interest at all in sexual relations, 21% a little, and only 14% had a moderate interest. For those women who maintained an interest in having sexual relations, 50% reported having pain or discomfort during intercourse. The majority of the patients did not suffer from non-satisfaction regarding their body or loss of masculinity or femininity in relation to their cancer or the treatment (Provencher et al., 2010).

4.5 Haematological cancer survivors

Survivors of haematological cancers including lymphoma do also experience sexual dysfunction especially those treated with bone marrow transplant. (Haematopoetic Stem Cell Transplant - HSCT). These patients usually receive cytotoxic chemotherapy and or whole body irradiation to suppress graft versus host reaction. Jean et al. (2009) in an extensive review of this aspect among survivors of HSCT noted that "these treatments impair the production of testosterone at least for the first year for males, and induce ovarian failure for most women. Effects are not solely gonadal. Treatments are known to permanently damage function of the hypothalamic-pituitary-gonadal axis. Luteinizing hormone (LH) is elevated in most female survivors and normal in most males. Follicle stimulating hormone is elevated in over 90% of females and most males. Most females have primary ovarian failure with consequent low endogenous oestrogen levels, and vaginal tissue atrophy is a risk. Chronic GVHD (Graft Versus Host Disease) may also contribute to vaginal introital stenosis and mucosal changes that contribute to dyspareunia, vaginal irritation, and increased sensitivity of genital tissues. Male sexual problems have been attributed to gonadal and cavernosal arterial insufficiency with resulting libido and erectile dysfunction." These reactions are mostly noted with alkylating agents class of cytotoxic drugs.

The lymphomas (Hodgkin's lymphoma [HL] and non-Hodgkin's lymphoma [NHL]) are among the most common cancers affecting men under 45 years. Survival rates are now excellent, but treatment is associated with a number of side effects including sexual dysfunction with potential implications for compromised quality of life (QoL). A study was carried out to address (i) the prevalence of sexual dysfunction among lymphoma survivors relative to the general population, survivors of other cancers, and in survivors of HL and NHL; and (ii) relationships between sexual functioning and disease and treatment, demographic, and psychological variables. Sexual function was found to be compromised relative to the general population, better than testicular cancer survivors, and worse than leukemia survivors. Depression was consistently associated with sexual dysfunction. There was evidence that chemotherapy, relapse, reduced testosterone levels, older age at survey, and worse physical QoL were associated with worse sexual function (Arden-Close et al., 2011). Another study found out that sexual problems were commonly reported by HL survivors, with 54.2% reporting decreased sexual activity and 41.4% reporting decreased interest. In the long term, this study did not show any difference in sexual function in long term survivors compared with the general population (Reclitis et al., 2010). However in another study on male lymphoma using Brief Sexual Function Index (BSFI) questionnaire, survivors had a mean age at survey of 47.4 years, the mean duration of follow-up was 14.8 years, and 79% lived in committed relationships. All BSFI domain scores decreased significantly with age. Lymphoma survivors also had low testosterone and/or elevated LH and had lower BSFI scores than survivors with normal gonadal hormones. Multivariate analyses showed that increasing age, more emotional distress, poor physical health, and low testosterone and/or elevated LH were significantly associated with reduced sexual function within the lymphoma group. Lymphoma survivors had significantly lower BSFI domain scores than did controls on erection, ejaculation, and sexual satisfaction (Kiserud et al., 2009). Erectile dysfunction has also been reported in 61% of lymphoma survivors assessed at least two years after treatment. (Aksoy et al., 2008). An earlier report found that chemotherapy for Hodgkin's disease produces ovarian failure in young women. The consequences of this are emotional distress, sexual dysfunction, and the disruption of families and friendships. These side effects of cytotoxic therapy had developed in 25 of 41 patients, among whom retrospective study was conducted (Chapman et al., 1979). Chemotherapy for Hodgkin's disease in that era however consisted of largely alkylating agents. Current combinations may not have such marked effects on ovarian function.

4.6 Central nervous system survivors

Survivors of brain tumours also experience sexual dysfunction. Neuroendocrine disturbances in anterior pituitary hormone secretion are common following radiation damage to the hypothalamic-pituitary (H-P) axis, the severity and frequency of which correlate with the total radiation dose delivered to the H-P axis and the length of follow-up. The somatotropic axis is the most vulnerable to radiation damage and GH deficiency remains the most frequently seen endocrinopathy. With low radiation doses (<30 Gy) GH deficiency usually occurs in isolation in about 30% of patients, while with radiation doses of 30-50 Gy, the incidence of GH deficiency can reach 50-100% and long-term gonadotropin, TSH and ACTH deficiencies occur in 20-30, 3-9 and 3-6% of patients, respectively. With higher dose cranial irradiation (>60 Gy) or following conventional irradiation for pituitary tumours (30-50 Gy), multiple hormonal deficiencies occur in 30-60% after 10 years of follow-up. Precocious puberty can occur after radiation doses of <30 Gy in girls only, and in both sexes equally with a radiation dose of 30-50 Gy. Hyperprolactinaemia, due to hypothalamic damage is mostly seen in young women after high dose cranial irradiation and is usually subclinical. H-P dysfunction is progressive and irreversible and can have an adverse impact on growth, body image, sexual function and quality of life. Regular testing is advised to ensure timely diagnosis and early hormone replacement therapy (Dalzy and Shalet, 2009). A prospective trial of the methods of sexual rehabilitation of 31 men with pituitary tumours has shown that therapy with testosterone and chorionic gonadotropin effectively corrects hypogonadism and sexual disorders. In insufficient efficacy, normalization of sexual function is achieved with tadalafil. Both methods of treatment had no negative effect on the size of the prostatic gland and PSA level except 2 patients with somatotropinoma on testosterone. In the course of chorionic gonadotropin treatment pituitary tumour increased in size in 3 patients (Rozhivanov & Kurbatov 2010). There is a case report of a 39-year-old patient with a history of high-grade anaplastic astrocytoma who presented to the Sexual Health Program at the Memorial Sloan-Kettering Cancer Center complaining of vaginal discharge and several months of amenorrhea. Although the patient was administered extensive aggressive antineoplastic treatments, her disease rapidly progressed. She was found to have mild vaginal atrophy and had improved sexual function after treatment which consisted of intravaginal non-hormonal moisturizers and vaginal lubricants, counselling, and sexual education (Krychman et al.,2004).

4.7 Survivors of sarcoma

Sarcomas of soft tissues and bones/ cartilages are usually treated with surgery (if possible depending on the site), radiotherapy and sometimes with chemotherapy consisting of vincristine, cyclophosphamde, doxorubicine with or without actinomycine D. Chemotherapy especially cyclophosphamide has been reported to be associated with low sperm count and raised follicle stimulating hormones in males . Exposure before puberty was not found to be protective and infertility was associated with high doses of cyclophosphamide. (Kenny et al., 2001) Total sacrectomy and reconstruction for patients with osteosarcoma, chondrosarcoma, giant cell tumour and chordoma in the sacral region is associated with high degree of sexual dysfunction likely due to disruption of the nerves around the site. (Wuisman et al., 2000)

4.8 Head and neck cancer survivors

Survivors of head and neck cancers also have sexual dysfunction. In a study involving 55 participants, eighty-five percent showed interest in sex. Fifty-eight percent were satisfied with their current sexual partner and 49% were satisfied with their current sexual functioning. Majority reported arousal problems, 58% did not participate in sexual intercourse, and 58% had orgasmic problems. Most patients were not depressed. There was no correlation between sexual functioning and performance status or severity of disfigurement. Patients younger than 65 years of age had more advanced disease, lower performance status and significantly poorer sexual functioning; those older than 65 years were more satisfied with their sexual partner and current sexual functioning (Monga et al, 1997).

Study instruments used in studies among head and neck cancer patients include Derogatis Sexual Function Scale, EORTIC QLQ H&N 37 sexual subscale

A quality of life studies among head and neck cancer survivors has been carried out at the Radiotherapy Department of The University College Hospital Ibadan Nigeria by the author. The aim of the study was to compare the quality of life pre treatment with quality of life at least 9 months post treatment of head and neck cancer patients seen at the centre. The materials and methods used included the assessment and evaluation of head and neck cancer patients that presented for treatment. All patients evaluated had histological confirmation of their conditions .Those with ECOG performance status greater than 2 or for palliative treatment were excluded as well as patients that were HIV positive. To study the sexuality component, The EORTIC H&N QLQ 35 questionnaire was used. There are only 2 questions that relate to the sexuality domain in the instrument and these are questions:

29. Have you felt less interest in sex? And 30. Have you felt less sexual enjoyment? These were assessed on a 4 point Likert scale as follows:

Not at all	A little	Quite a bit	Very much
1	2	3	4

The questionnaires were administered before commencement of treatment and at least 9 months after treatment during follow up visits.

A total of 100 patients were evaluated. The characteristics of the patients are presented in table 2.

Age group distributions	
Age group (yrs)	
16-25	13(13%)
26-35	9(9%)
36-45	20(20%)
46-55	16(16%)
56-65	24(24%)
66-75	0 (0%)
76-85	18(18%)
Sex:	
Male	58(58%)
Female	42(42%)
Marital status:	
Single	21(21%)
Married	70(70%)
Widow/widower	9(9%)
Level of Education:	
Primary	6(6%)
Secondary	38(38%)
Tertiary	31(31%)
None	25(25%)

Table 2. Head and Neck Quality of Life (Sex) studies : Patients' characteristics. (N=100)

The overall mean age was 49.86 years with a range of 18-85 years and Standard Deviation (SD) = 17.48. Mean age for males = 51.59 years, range = 19-85 years and SD = 16.93 while mean age for females = 47.60 years with a range of 18-85 years and SD = 18.39. The pre-treatment and post treatment scores are presented in table 3

	Pre- treatment scores	post treatment scores	Std Deviation	p-value
Overall (mean)	38.6	49.8	18.00	0.00
Male	35.0	46.2	31.38	
Female	42.2	53.9	28.70	0.21
Stage				
1/11		44.0	29.67	
111/1V		50.3	30.56	0.47
Disease Sites				
Oral cavity	40	44		
Nasopharynx:	49	58		
Oropharynx :	50	53		
Larynx:	36	50		
Sino-nasal region	44	60		
Salivary gland:	32	36		
Thyroid gland	15	41		

Table 3. Head and Neck Quality of Life (Sex) Scores (N=100)

These results show that there were reduction in sexual functioning in all the patients after treatment for head and neck cancers and these were noticed with all cancer sites. Survivors of cancers of the Sino-nasal region experienced the highest sexual problems followed by those with laryngeal cancers among the core head and neck cancer patients. Survivors of thyroid cancer however had the highest score of sexual dysfunction and it is better considered separately as endocrine cancers since hypothyroidism can result in sexual dysfunction. Patients with advanced diseases (stages 111 &1V) experienced more sexual problems than those with early diseases (stages 1 & 11).[P value 0.47] This is similar to earlier reports by Monga et al.,(1997) who reported poorer sexual function among patients with advanced disease which was more in those 65 years and above. The result also shows that the effect was more on females than males (P value 0.21). This may probable be due to the use of chemotherapy which may have more effects on the hormonal status of the female patients. Some chemotherapy agents affect the ovaries leading to reduction in the amount of circulating oestrogen. This leads to reduced sexual functions. Ovarian failure occurs most often in women who are above 35 years of age after chemotherapy (Schover, 2008).

The reported changes in sexuality is important because the mean age of these patients was 49 years which means that these patients are relatively young and therefore sexually active, as this is an important social aspect for many of them.

This analysis gives an indication that these patients have sexual issues following treatment. These issues need to be addressed by care givers. More detailed study focussing on sexuality of survivors using questionnaires that can evaluate specific aspects of sexual function is required for better assessment and management of survivors of head and neck cancers in this environment.

4.9 Lung cancer survivors

Sexual problems exist among survivors of lung cancer. A report noted that sexual concerns were common, with 52% of patients reporting at least mild sexual concerns and were stable. Sexual concerns were significantly associated with physical and emotional symptoms. Particularly strong relationships were found between sexual concerns and shortness of breath and emotional distress. Age moderated the relationship between both fatigue and shortness of breath and sexual concerns. Gender moderated the relationship between emotional distress and sexual concerns. Self-reported sexual concerns were noted to be common in people with lung cancer, are stable, and are related significantly to physical and emotional symptoms. Age and gender influenced the distress associated with sexual symptoms in this population.(Reese et al., 2011)

4.10 Management of sexual dysfunction

It is important that sexual issues be looked into among cancer patients especially after treatment. During the course of the disease, lots of issues like anxiety concerning the disease and its treatment, financial issues, employment related issues and other social issues may affect sexual health of the patients. Those who have completed their treatment will be free from many other co- founding problems and sexual issues will come to the fore. These have to be addressed as part of the patients' management. It is also pertinent to note that these issues vary in intensity with respect to duration of survival hence periodic reassessment needed for necessary adjustments in pattern of care.

4.10.1 Assessment

Cancer survivors should be assessed for sexual dysfunction before treatment and as soon as they are clinically stable. It is important to know the pre treatment sexual functioning of the individual as this varies from person to person. This baseline information will also enable the health personnel to assess the degree of variation ascribable to the disease and its treatment. Anxiety and depression associated with the illness should be identified and managed before addressing sexual concerns. There is also need to distinguish cancer patients with sexual difficulties and concomitant psychosocial stressors (*e.g.*, financial, familial, occupational, marital). These latter difficulties could disrupt the range, frequency, enjoyment, or importance of sexual activity for cancer patients as they sometimes do for healthy individuals.) from those without additional stressors, allowing more specific etiologic associations to be identified

Discussions on survivors sexual health can be commenced using some tools like:-

PLISSIT model—Permission, Limited Information, Specific Suggestions and Intensive Therapy. This model involves four stages to guide the assessment and treatment of sexual dysfunction. The first stage, permission, involves providing the patient with an opportunity to discuss sexual problems or concerns. Limited information involves the provision of general information about the sexual problem and options for intervention. Specific suggestions would include detailed discussions about treatment options and techniques that could be used to improve sexual activity. Intensive Therapy usually involves referral to a specialist. This model can be used to systematically guide the healthcare professional through the evaluation of sexual dysfunction and the provision of information. (Stead 2004) ALARM model- Activity, Libido, Arousal, Resolution, Medical information. Communication has to be initiated by the health care personnel with the patients concerning the above aspects of their sexual lives in order to establish possible areas of intervention. PLEASURE model -Partner, Lovemaking, Emotions Attitude, Symptoms, Understanding, Reproduction Energy.

BETTER model- Bring up the topic, Explain that sexuality is an important aspect of quality of life and should be discussed, Tell patients that there are resource s available to address concerns or problems, Timing is important, offer discussions and let them know you are available anytime, Educate patients and families how treatment can impact sexuality, Record discussions , assessment, interventions and outcomes (Audette & Waterman 2010).

These tools can be applied for general screening of patients for sexual dysfunction and it is recommended that this assessment should be done periodically to monitor the patients. Detailed diagnostic tools could then be applied in those with established problems for more specific diagnosis based on disease site and patients characteristics. A list of some other tools that can be used to assess various aspects of sexual dysfunction is provided in table 4..

4.10.2 Treatment

Some physical therapy like exercises can help in the treatment of some forms of sexual dysfunction as part of general well being resulting from exercise. Specific exercises like pelvic floor exercises can promote relaxation and help in relieving dyspareunia following treatment of some gynaecological malignancies. Intercourse should be encouraged at least three times per week following pelvic irradiation in women. Alternatively, vaginal dilators of fingers can be used at least three times per week for ten minutes to keep the vaginal canal patent. This is also useful towards follow up examinations (Borduka & Sun 2006). Pharmacological agents like non steroidal lubricants for women are also available for those experiencing vaginal dryness. Psychological therapy especially by specialists can improve the situation. Hormonal replacements may be useful especially in some hormone associated conditions like following treatment for pituitary tumours and other endocrine malignancies.

Name of Questionnaire	Author(s)	Original language
Arizona Sexual Experience Scale	Gelenberg, A.	English
Brief Index for Sexual Functioning for women (BISF-F)	Rosen ,R.	English
Brief Sexual Function Index (BSFI)	O'Leary, M.	English
Changes in Sexual Functioning Questionnaire (CSFQ)- F & M Components	Clayton ,A	English
Derogatis Index for Sexual Functioning (DISF) M & F	Derogatis, L	English
Erectile dysfunction Inventory of Treatment Satisfaction (EDITS)	Altof S Et al., for Pfizer Inc	English
Erectile Dysfunction Quality of Life ED EQOL	Mac Donagh	English
Erectile Dysfunction Question (EDQ)	Araujo, A.	English
Female Sexual Desire Profile (FSDP)	Nillson ,A.	English
Female Sexual Distress Scale (FSDS)	Derogatis, L.	English
Female Sexual Distress Scale (FSDS)- Revised 2005	Derogatis, L.	English
Female Sexual Encounter Profile - adapted (FSEPa)	Ferguson D.	English
Female Sexual Function Questionnaire (FSFQ)	Quirk, F	English
Female Sexual Function Index (FSFI)	Rosen ,R & Ferguson D	English
International Index of Erectile Function (IERF)	Rosen, R for Pfizer Inc	English
International Index of Erectile Function (IERF)- Partner Diary	Rosen ,R. For Pfizer Inc	English
Inventory of Treatment satisfaction (ITS)	Althof et al.	English
Mc coy Sexuality Questionnaire (MFSQ)	Mc Coy, N.	English
MOS Sexual Function Module (MOS-SEXUAL)	Ware Dr.	English
Psychosexual Daily Questionnaire (PDQ)	Wang, C.	English
Sexual Activity Questionnaire (SEXACQ)	Fallowfield L	English
Sexual Function Index (SFI)	O'Leary	English
Sexual Life Quality Questionnaire (SLQQ)	Lass, S.	English
Sexual Satisfaction Module (SEXTES)	Testa, M.	English

Table 4. Specific Questionnaires: Sexuality. Adapted from Mapi Institute (n.d.)

5. Conclusion

The prevalence of sexual dysfunction among cancer survivors is high and the extent varies according to years of survival, disease site, age and sex of the patients. It should therefore be borne in mind that almost all oncology patients have sexual issues. There is need for improvement in the routine assessment of sexual functions among cancer survivors. To enhance this, training on basic assessment techniques including communication should be undergone by all those who partake in the care of cancer patients. There is also need for increased training in management of sexual issues and management techniques should be improved upon through further research for effectiveness.

6. Acknowledgement

I wish to acknowledge the assistance of Dr Adamu Bojude, Departmant of Radiation Oncology, University College Hospital Ibadan Nigeria for his assistance on the study on sexual dysfunction of Head and Neck Cancer survivors seen at the department of Radiation Oncology, University College Hospital Ibadan Nigeria.

7. References

Alfano, C.; Smith, A.; Irwin, M.; Bowen D.; Sorensen B.; Reeve B & Tiernan A (2007). Physical activity,long term symptoms and physical health related quality of life among breast cancer survivors: A prospective analysis. *Journal of Cancer Survival* Vol.1 No. 2 (Dec 2007)pp. 116-128.

Aksoy S, Harputluoglu H, Kilickap S, Dincer M, Dizdar O, Akdogan B, Ozen H, Erman M & Celik I (2007). Erectile dysfunction in successfully treated lymphoma patients. *SupportCare Cancer.* 2008 Mar; Vol.16 No.3 (Mar 2008): pp.291-297.

Andersen L, & NF (1983). Psychosexual adjustment following pelvic exenteration. *Obstet Gynecol.* No (1983) pp.61:331–338

Andersen L.(1990) How cancer affects sexual functioning. *Oncology (Williston Park).* Vol.4 No.6 (June1990) pp:81-88

Andersen, L. (1985).Sexual Functioning Morbidity Among Cancer Survivors: Current Status and Future Research Directions *Cancer.* Vol. 55 No.8 (April 1985)pp 1835–1842

Aqua H, Jayne D, Eu K & Seow-Choen K (2002). Bladder and sexual dysfunction following laparascopically assisted and conventional open meso rectal resection for cancer. *British Journal of Surgery* vol. 89 2002 pp 1551-1556.

Arden-Close E, Eiser C& Pacey A. (2011) Sexual Functioning in Male Survivors of Lymphoma: A Systematic Review. *J Sex Med.* No 16 (Feb2011) pp.1000-.1111

Audette C and Waterman J. The Sexual Health of Women after Gynaecologic Malignancy (2010) *Journal of Midwifery and Womens Health* Vol 55 No. 4 (July 2010) pp 357-362.

Barni, S. & Mondin, R. (1997). Sexual dysfunction in treated breast cancer patients. *Annals of Oncology* Vol. 8, (1997) pp. 149-153

Bober, S. Reclitis , C. Campbell, E., Park, E. Kutner J. Najita J. & Diller , l. (2009). Caring for cancer survivors. *Cancer* Vol.115 No. S18 (Sept 2009) pp. 4409-4418.

Bonini-Colmano M.; Molnar S.; Salvano L.; Molina G.; Arevelo M.; Di Marco P.; Rizzi M. & Dibersarsky C. (2007) Sexual dysfunction in patients with cancer. *Journal of Clinical Oncology* 2007 ASCO Annual meeting proceedings Part 1 Vol 25 No. 18S (June supplement 2007) Abstract 19653.

Borduka D & Sun C (2006). Sexual function after gynaecological cancer . *Obstetrics Gynaeco clin of N Am* No 33 (,2006) pp.621-630

Bukovic D.; Fajdic, J.; Argovic Z.; Kaufmann M.; Hojsak I. & Stanceric T (2005). Sexual dysfunction in breast cancer survivors. *Onkologie* vol. 28 No. 1 (2005) pp. 29-34

Carmack-Taylor l, Basen-Engquist k, Shinn E and Bodurka D (2004) Predictors of sexual functioning in ovarian cancer patients. *Journal of Clinical Oncology* No 22 (2004) pp. 881-889

Carter J, Goldfrank D, Schover LR (2011). Simple strategies for vaginal health promotion in cancer survivors. *J Sex Med.* Vol.8 No.2 (Feb 2011) pp.549-559

Cella D, Fallowfield L, Barker P, Cuzick J, Locker &, Howell A (2006). Quality of life of postmenopausal women in the ATAC ("Arimidex", tamoxifen, alone or in combination) trial after completion of 5 years' adjuvant treatment for early breast cancer. *Breast Cancer Res Treat. No.*100 (2006) pp.273–84

Chapman R, Sutcliffe S & Malpas J (1979) Cytotoxic-induced ovarian failure in Hodgkin's disease Effects on sexual function. *JAMA.* .26; Vol.242 No.17 (Oct 1979):pp.1882-1884.

Darzy K&, Shalet S (2009) . Hypopituitarism following Radiotherapy Revisited *Endocr Dev* No.15 (2009) pp 1-24.

Fallowfield L, Cella D, Cuzick J, Francis S, Locker G & Howell A. (2004). Quality of life of postmenopausal women in the Arimidex, Tamoxifen, Alone or in Combination (ATAC) Adjuvant Breast Cancer Trial. *J Clin Oncol. Vol* 22, (2004) pp. 4261–71

Fallowfield LJ, Bliss JM, Porter LS, et al (2006). Quality of life in the intergroup exemestane study: a randomized trial of exemestane versus continued tamoxifen after 2 to 3 years of tamoxifen in postmenopausal women with primary breast cancer. *J Clin Oncol.* No.249 (2006) PP. 910–917s

Ganz PA, Desmond KA, Belin TR, et al (1999). Predictors of sexual health in women after a breast cancer diagnosis. *Journal of Clinical Oncolology* No. *17.*(1999) pp.2371-2380

Ganz, P.; Rowland J.; Desmond, K.; Meyerowitz B.; & Wyatt G (1998). Life after breast cancer: Understanding women's health related quality of life and sexual functioning. *Journal of Clinical Oncology* No. 16 (1998) pp 501-514

Ganz PA, Coscarelli A, Fred C, et al (1996) Breast cancer survivors: psychosocial concerns and quality of life. *Breast Cancer Res Treat.* No.38 (1996) pp.183-199.

Gilbert, S. Dunn, R B. Hollenbeck, J. Montie, J. Lee, C, Wood D. & Wei J. (2010). Development and Validation of the Bladder Cancer Index:A Comprehensive, Disease Specific Measure of Health Related Quality of Life in Patients With Localized Bladder Cancer *Journal of Urology* Vol.183 No 5 (2010) pp. 1764-1769

Green M, Naumann R, Elliot M, et al(2000).: Sexual dysfunction following vulvectomy. *Gynecol Oncol* 2000, No.77 (2000) pp.73–77.

Greenfield M, Walters J, Coleman R, Hancock B, Snowden J, Shalet S, DeRogatis L &, Ross R. (2010) Quality of life, self-esteem, fatigue, and sexual function in young men after cancer: a controlled cross-sectional study. *Cancer.* Vol.116 No.6 (March 2010) pp.1592-601.

Hartmann,J. Albrecht C, Schmoll H, Kuczyk M, Kollmannsberger C & Bokemeyer C (1999) . Long-term effects on sexual function and fertility after treatment of testicular cancer. *British Journal of Cancer* Vol 80 No.5/6 (1999), pp. 801–807

Joly F.; Degrendel A.; Guizard A.;(2010). Quality of life after radiotherapy for prostate cancer. *Cancer Radiother.* 2010 Oct Vol.14 No.6-7 Oct (2010) pp.519-25.

Kenney L, Laufer M, Grant F, Grier H& Diller L.(2001).High risk of infertility and long term gonadal damage in males treated with high dose cyclophosphamide for sarcoma during childhood. *Cancer.* 2001 Feb Vol.91 No.3 (Feb 2001):pp.613-621.

Kiserud C, Schover L, Dahl A, Fossay A, BiA ¸ro T, Loge J, Holte H, Yuan Y, & Fossay S (2009). Do male lymphoma survivors have impaired sexual function? *J Clin Oncol.* Vol.27 No.35 (Dec 2009) pp. 6019-26.

Krychman M, Amsterdam A, Carter J, Castiel M & DeAngelis L. Brain cancer and sexual health: a case report. *Palliat Support Care.* Vol.2 No.3 (Sep 2004): pp.315-318.

Land SR, Wickerham DL, Costantino JP, et al.(2006) Patient-reported symptoms and quality of life during treatment with tamoxifen or raloxifene for breast cancer prevention: the NSABP Study of Tamoxifen and Raloxifene (STAR) P-2 trial. *Jama.* Vol.295 (2006) pp.2742-2751

Lindau, S. Anderson, D & Gavrilova, N (2007) Sexual Morbidity in Very long-term Survivors of Vaginal and Cervical Cancer: A Comparison to National Norms *Gynecol Oncol.* Vol 106 No.2 (August 2007) pp. 413–418.

Lindley C,Vasa S, Sawyer WT, et al. (1998) Quality of life and preferences for treatment following systemic adjuvant therapy for early stage breast cancer. *Journal of Clinical Oncology.* No *16 (*1998) pp.1380-1387.

Ntekim, A.; Nuhu F. & Campbell O (2009). Breast cancer in young females in Ibadan Nigeria. *African Health Sciences* Vol. 9 No. 4 (2009) pp 242-246

Melisko M.;bGoldman M.& Rugo S. (2010). Amelioration of sexual adverse effects of the early breast cancer patient. *Journal of Cancer Survival* Vol.4 No. 3 (Sept 2010)pp. 247-255

Mapi Institute (n.d.) Sexuality in *Specific Questionnaires* Accessed June 26, 2011, <Available http. www. Mapi-institute.com/ component/content/article/6-list/135- specific-questionnaires-sexuality

Monga U, Tan G, Ostermann H, Monga TN(1997.) .Sexuality in head and neck cancer patients *Arch Phys Med Rehab* Vol.78 No.3: (Mar 1997) pp.298-304

Morrow P .(2011). Long term effects of the diagnosis and treatment of breast cancer upon young breast cancer survivors. *Journal of Clinical Oncology* Vol. 29. No. 15S Part 1 of 11 (May 2011) p 560S.

Ofman, S. (1995). Preservation of function in genitor-urinary cancers: psychosexual and psychosocial issues. *Cancer Investigations,* vol.13.No. 1 (1995) pp. 125-131

Park,, E.; Bober, S.; Campbell, E.; Recklitis, C.; Kutner, J.& Diller, L (2009) General Internist Communication about Sexual Function with Cancer Survivors *J Gen Intern Med.* No 24 Suppl 2 (Nov.2009) pp. 407–411.

Passik S, Newman M.; Brennan M. & Tunkel R. (1995) Predictors of psychological distress, sexual dysfunction and physical functioning among women with upper extremity lymphedema related to breast cancer *Psycho Oncology* Vol 4 No.4,(1995)pp. 255-263

Recklitis C, Sanchez Varela V, Ng A, Mauch P & Bober S (2010). Sexual functioning in long-term survivors of Hodgkin's lymphoma. *Psycho -oncology.* Vol.19 No.11 (Nov 2010):pp.1229-1233.

Reese J, Shelby R & Abernethy A. (2011).Sexual concerns in lung cancer patients: an examination of predictors and moderating effects of age and gender. *Support Care Cance*r. 2011 Jan;Vol.19 No.1 (Jan 2011):pp.161- 165.

Rozhivanov R&, Kurbatov D (2010). Sexual function rehabilitation of men with pituitary tumors. *Urologiia* Vol. 4 No. 48 (Jul-Aug.2010) pp 50-53. .

Sawyna Provencher S; Oehler, C.Lovertu S, Jolicoeur, M Fortin, B. & Donath D. Quality of life and tumor control after short split-course chemoradiation for anal canal carcinoma *Radiat Oncol.* 2010; Vol 5: No.41(May 2010) pp 1000-1186.

Schover L (2008) Premature ovarian failure and its consequences: Vasomotor symptoms, sexuality and fertility. *J Clin Oncol* No.26,(2008) pp.753-758.

Speer, J.; Hillenberg, B.; Sugrue, D.; Blacker, C.; Kresge C.; Decker, V.; Zakalik D. & Decker, D. (2005) Study of sexual functioning determinants in breast cancer survivors. *The Breast Journal* Vol. 11 No. 6 (2005) pp. 440-4471.

Sprangers M, Taal B, Aaronson N and Velde, A (2007). Quality of life in colorectal cancer. Stoma versus non stoma patients. *Diseases of Colon and Rectum* , vol 38,No.4 (2007) pp. 361-369

Stead, L. (2003) .Sexual dysfunction after treatment for gynaecologic and breast malignancies. *Current Opinion in Obstetrics & Gynecology.* Vol. 15 No. 1 (Feb 2003) - pp 57-61

Stead L (2004). Sexual function after treatment for gynaecological malignancy *Curr Opin Oncol* No 16 (2004) pp :492–495.

Steel J.;Hess S,; Tunke L .;& Carr B Chopra K (2005). Sexual Functioning in Patients with Hepatocellular Carcinoma. *Cancer* Vol 104 No 10 (Nov 2005) pp 2234-2243

Thors C.; Broeckel, J.; & Jacobson P. (2001). Sexual functioning in breast cancer survivors. *Cancer Control* Vol. 8 No. 5 (Oct 2001) pp.442-448

Thuesen B, Andreasson B,& Bock JE: (1992) Sexual function and somapsychic reactions after local excision of vulval intra-epithelial neoplasia. *Acta Obstet Gynaecol Scand,* No.71 (1992) pp.126–128.

Tiv M, Puyraveau M, Mineur L, Calais G, Maingon P, Bardet E, Mercier M & Bosset J. (2010) Long-term quality of life in patients with rectal cancer treated with preoperative (chemo)-radiotherapy within a randomized trial. *Cancer Radiother.*;Vol.14 No.6-7 (Oct 2010) pp.530-534.

Wuisman P, Lieshout O, Sugihara S & van Dijk M.(2000). Total sacrectomy and reconstruction: oncologic and functional outcome. *Clin Orthop Relat Res*. 2000 Dec;No.381 (Dec 2000):pp.192-203.

Yi, J. & Syrjala, K.(2009) Sexuality after Hematopoietic Stem Cell Transplantation *Cancer J*. Vol.15 No.1 (2009) pp. 57–64.

4

Sexual Rehabilitation of People with Physical Disabilities: Sexuality and Spinal Injury

Ana Cláudia Bortolozzi Maia
Universidade Estadual Paulista Júlio de Mesquita Filho- UNESP
Brasil

1. Introduction

This article intends to discuss the sexuality of people with physical deficiencies, focusing on sexual rehabilitation. It is based on a comprehensive review intending to explore some fundamental concepts, theoretical reflections and practices in the text about this thematic dealing with: (a) Concepts about sexuality and disability, (b) The sexuality of people with physical disabilities and (c) The sexual rehabilitation of people with a spinal injury.

1.1 The concept of sexuality and disabilities

Thinking about sexual rehabilitation means thinking about affective, emotional and sexual restructuring of the individual using the vast concept of sexuality defended here as a base, according to Foucault (1988), as a social and historical concept.

Sexual practices, corporal and sexual biological expressions are expressed in difficult cultures and under different social and economic conditions. Therefore sexuality refers to a comprehensive phenomenon of human eroticism, considering the organic, psychological and social issues. Additionally, its expression is vast and widespread and depends on different cultural contexts and historical moments (Anderson, 2000; Bozon, 2004; Blackburn, 2002; Daniels, 1981; Maia, 2010; 2011).

In this sense, even though the phenomenon of the sexual response can be described physiologically, it is important to remember that its expression depends on psychosocial representations. The perceptions of desire, excitation and orgasm, have to do with the way in which these pleasurable corporal experiences were received throughout their life and how they are considered in different societies.

Foucault (2002) proposes that sexuality, including the instinctual direction of the desire, the representation of the body, gender, diverse sexual practices, is constructed from a combination of social, cultural, historical and discursive institutions mediated by the knowledge-power discourse. This social discourse regarding sexuality generates norms that should be controlled based on the idea that it would be normal or abnormal. These models considered as defining normality standards involve issues such as gender, race, ethnicity, educational level and economic among other questions that always involve power (Stoller, 1998; Weeks, 1999).

Therefore, sexuality, understood as historical and cultural phenomenon, reflects the concepts, values and parameters about "normal" and "pathological" that set themselves in contexts where sexual practices occur (Maia, 2010; Stoller, 1998). The sexuality considered "normal" contains certain sexual patterns, which in our society, are related to questions like: being heterosexual, having a thin and skinny body, having sexual and reproductive health and having a sexually functional response.

We want "normal" sexuality based on these standards, believing that if we're "adequate", we'll feel pleasure and happiness (Maia, 2009). It's important to point out that not corresponding to certain sexual standards imposed by societies do not make somebody asexual, but it can result in fragmented sexual expression and cause unhappiness and social maladjustment. Thus, functional and dysfunctional social practices reflect a notion of normalcy and ideology.

Another important concept is disability as a social construction, because the organic and functional limits of the human body correspond to disadvantageous representations when society is based on the notion of productivity and competitiveness (Aranha, 1995; Amaral, 1995; Marques, 1997; Omote, 1999; Ross, 1998; Tomasini, 1998). I am referring to the exclusion of those who possess unequal conditions for productivity, such as the elderly and people with deficiencies.

"Disability" refers to a series of general conditions that limit someone's life biologically, psychologically or socially throughout their development (Maia, 2006). It emerges as something that separates the subject from normalcy; it is considered a deviation, placed in a condition of "defectiveness", "insufficiency" and "imperfection". The way in which such differences are judged reflects how we conceive what is and what should be normal and healthy (Amaral, 1995; Maia, 2009; Omote, 1999; Tomasini, 1998; Siebers, 2008; Sorrentino, 1990).

Therefore, even though the disability and difference appears in a biological body or atypical behavior, it can only be considered a "disability" as a social phenomenon, that is out of the subject's control, and not intrinsic to them. It is society that judges and classifies that as a disability or not, and establishes the parameters of what it means to be host that difference in comparison to everybody else (Amaral, 1995; Aranha, 1995; Omote, 1999). That judgment results in stigmatization (Goffman, 1988).

Generally, social opinion places disability as a condition of disadvantage based on socially undesirable attributes. It's evident that disability isn't just a mere detail, but a label, a stamp that makes its subject deal with a series of difficulties, a constant fight for equal rights, favorable conditions in order to be a conscientious citizen (Maia, 2006; 2011). Siebers (2008) claims that disability is a minority identity that has been historically seen as a condition that's a target for medical intervention, but should be understood as a product of society, constructed in the context where it manifests itself. The disability isn't a personal and individual problem, but a social and collective one (Edwards, 1997; Maia, 2011; Mitchell & Synder, 1997; Pristley, 2001; Siebers, 2008).

Thus, we can grasp that the concept of disability is created and maintained by society. That is, the social belief about the phenomenon, in this case, the whole idea is therefore social, cultural and historical (Amaral, 1995; Marques, 1997; Omote, 1999; Ribas, 1998; Siebers, 2008; Tomasini, 1998). According to Aranha (1995, p.69) "those who don't correspond to the efficiency/production parameters, will naturally be worthless by becoming contradictions to the system exposing its limitations".

Above all, it's because of this, that it is necessary to understand - and reflect - about the prevailing concept in relation to disabled people and disabilities and deficiencies in our society at this historic moment. Certainly, despite the advance represented by the inclusive paradigm even though in practice, there aren't any guarantees, of accomplishing the best

possibilities of developing a life healthy and worthy of a conscientious citizen in relation to education, work, and also sexuality (Maia, 2006; 2011).
It's possible to deduce that one of the great barriers to inclusion is the stigma, and this, as in all prejudice, also disregards diversity with respect to sexuality. Considering sexuality and disability as social conditions, think about the biological body in terms that sexual rehabilitation results in questioning which social meanings are subjective components and which are feelings of personal inadequacy.

1.2 The sexuality of people with physical disabilities

The capacity to love and be loved and the erotic desires that are inherent to human beings are preserved under any limitation; that is to say that no human being loses their sexuality even when they have certain motor or physiological restrictions. Many times social prejudice turns sexuality impossible in people with disabilities.
"It's necessary to be clear that sexuality is independent - or not - on the existence of incapacity; in other words, sexuality is inherent to human beings; the differences occur in the manifestation of the sexual activity, which can be modified in some cases. Disability isn't definitely synonymous to asexuality or sexual problematic" (Pinel, 1999, p.214-215).
The greatest difficulties in the expression of sexuality in the case of people with physical disabilities refer to social questions more than to organic limitation. The main questions are prejudice, misinformation, discrimination, inability, lack of adequate sexual orientation, insufficient or inadequate process of sex education by their Family, disbelief in the capacity of disabled people to express their sentiments and sexual desires, values, and distorted ideas associated with physical disabilities (Blackburn, 2002; Pinel, 1999; Maia, 2006; 2011).
The sexuality of the disabled person is a multi-faceted phenomenon: economic, political, cultural and educational questions (Fróes, 2000; Maia, 2006). Additionally, people with a disability suffer the effects of beauty standards, perfection and happiness, especially when they are women. Many people with a disability incorporate the expectations of sexual standards and internalize the even more difficult task of reaching them, when the disability exists (França & Chaves, 2005; Louro, Faro & Chaves, 1997; Maia, 2011; Sorrentino, 1990; Werebe, 1984).
Authors such as Anderson and Kitchin (2000) have defended that the majority of day-to-day difficulties encountered by people with disabilities in relation to sexuality is caused by the failure of available education resources and services to provide them with clarification about the subject. According to Pinel (1999) the majority of people with disabilities reproduce a social image that can generate socialization problems related to deprivation of affection, emotional dependence and also difficulties in becoming adults capable of fighting for their rights including those related to sexuality.
So, the sexuality of people with disabilities is perceived in common sense–that reflects on work with teachers, diverse professional, and clients themselves and their family members - based on different myths. Some of these myths are: people with disabilities are asexual: they have no feelings, thoughts and sexual needs, people with disabilities have a hyper sexuality: their desires are uncontrollable and exacerbated, people with disabilities are unattractive, undesirable and unable to love and have a sexual relationship, people with disabilities are unable to enjoy *normal* sex and have sexual dysfunctions related to desire, excitement and orgasm, reproduction for people with disabilities is always problematic because people are infertile, have children with disabled or are unable to take care of them

(Andreson, 2000; Amaral, 1995; Baer, 2003; Giami, 2004; Kaufman, Silverberg & Odette, 2003; Maia, 2011; Maia & Ribeiro, 2010; Pinel, 1999; Salimene, 1995).

Those ideas are myths because they don't correspond to the truth. People with disabilities are always sexual beings, even though they might have some sort of physical or sexual limitation: they don't characterize themselves as asexual nor as hypersexual, their anxieties, necessities and desires are the same as those with healthy bodies. Additionally, possible problems in the sexual response phases, such as desire, excitement and orgasm are common in groups with and without disabilities. In both cases there are resources and behavioral technologies that can help overcome these obstacles, therefore the sex life of a person with a disability is not synonymous with incapacity and unhappiness.

Belief in these myths reveals a biased way of understanding the sexuality of disabled people as deviant from normal standards and it becomes an obstacle to love and to have sex for these who are stigmatized by the disability and because of this, clarifying these myths is a necessary task to minimize the prejudice that sustains and reproduces them (Maia & Ribeiro, 2010).

1.3 Sexual rehabilitation of people with spinal cord injuries

1.3.1 Spinal cord injury: Characteristics, etiology and prognosis

Spinal cord injury is a medical condition that severely affects various bodily functions, often causing motor paralysis, loss of sensibility in certain body parts and lack of bladder or bowel control. These symptoms may be temporary, but often are permanent (Ducharme & Gill, 1997). Spinal cord injury, therefore, is defined as a clinical condition that produces alteration in motor, sensory and neurovegetative functions, which also are reflected in profound psychological and social changes.

The spine consists of vertebrae superimposed on a regular basis, held together by ligaments and disposed on the center line of the posterior trunk. Its function is to hold the bones of the body and protect the spinal cord. The spine is divided into four regions - cervical, thoracic, lumbar and sacral. The spinal canal serves to protect the spinal cord, the roots of spinal nerves and the meninges (Baer, 2003; Cardoso, 2006).

To define the spinal cord injury it is important to consider the specific circumstances of each case, depending on the level and extent of injury. A neurological examination is able to evaluate the injury by determining the level of damage, whether it will result in paraplegia or quadriplegia and whether it is complete or incomplete. Cardoso (2006) explains:

"Thus, tetraplegia is defined as the loss or impairment of motor and/or sensory function in the cervical segments of the spinal cord caused by destruction of neural elements within the spinal canal resulting in a alteration of function of the upper and lower limbs, trunk and pelvic organs. (...) In turn paraplegia is defined as the loss or impairment of motor and/or sensory function in thoracic, lumbar or sacral spinal cord, because of the destruction of neural elements within the spinal canal. In paraplegia the upper limb function remains intact, but depending on the level of the injury, trunk, lower limbs and pelvic organs may be functionally impaired" (p.58).

Other issues arising from spinal cord injuries are secondary complications such as pressure ulcers, urinary infections, pain, spasticity, and obesity, problems that worsen with time (Salimene, 1995, Maia, 2011).

The causes of spinal cord injuries can be grouped into traumatic and non-traumatic. In the first group, the lesions occur in car accidents, falls, firearms, at work or in sports practice, etc.. In the second group are the medical conditions (spinal tumors, myelitis, scoliosis, multiple sclerosis, congenital malformations, spinal vascular accidents etc (Cardoso, 2006; Salimene, 1995, Maia, 2006).

Spinal cord injury affects mainly young male adults. It is rare among children and these data are similar in different countries (Baer, 2003; Pinel, 1999; Salimene, 1995). Moreover, the spinal segments that suffer most injuries are located between the cervical articulations. The severity of neurological impairment resulting from a spinal cord injury reflects the nature and magnitude of the violence of the injury, which may result from bending, compression, hyperextension and flexion-rotation against any region of the column where this impact operates (Cardoso, 2006).

Concerning these aspects, the prognosis will depend crucially on the area and the extent of injury. According to Cardoso (2006), considering the injuries in general, there is a mortality rate of 38% soon after the injury or the initial phase, due to respiratory or trophy disease. However, currently, the expectation of life of individuals affected by the injury has increased significantly.

1.3.2 The sexual response in people with spinal cord injury

Physical disabilities, especially those of the spinal cord, were total and partial paralysis, loss of motor functions and feeling in the legs (paraplegia), or in the legs, torso and arms (tetraplegia) can have direct implications on the sexual response mechanism. That is to say problems in the sexual phase (penile erection or vaginal lubrication) and even more in the orgasm and ejaculation phases. Depending on the level and extension of the spinal cord injury, some sexual response alterations are recurring, specially in men, where changes in ejaculation can occur (ejaculation lock) and in the erection (partial or complete erectile dysfunction or maintenance) and retrograde ejaculation (Baer, 2003; Cardoso, 2006; Ducharme & Gill, 1997; Maia, 2010, Maior, 1988; Pinel, 1999).

Sexual function consists of three levels, the psychic, gonadal, and neuromuscular, and for its manifestation to occur normally, good functioning and integration of these three levels are necessary (Maior 1988). Salimene (1995) says it's evident that spinal cord injuries accentuate physical and functional limitations, but that's not to say that there's necessarily going to be problems in relation to the overall sexual manifestation. According to Cardoso (2006), the limbic system and spinal cord centers constitute sexuality's neurological substrate, but this is influenced by cognitive and sociocultural mechanisms like fears, expectations and beliefs, and by personal evaluation of one's sexual response.

From a psychological point of view, sexual desire seems to be associated with cognitive activity and, from an organic viewpoint, it is related to cerebral activity, activity through the limbic system, influenced by testosterone. Desire is governed by many biological mechanisms in relation to availability and the subject's receptivity with the other that had psychological and social influence. In people with physical disabilities and spinal cord injuries, desire is a phase where they might or might not suffer alterations, especially arising from psychological and social issues, more than organic ones. It is common to hear between those with spinal cord injuries, that desire decreases after the lesion, what could be related to the lesion, but also to mechanisms that affect the nervous system and even reduced mobility, and spasticity and problems with intestinal and bladder control. On the other hand, physical intimacy, even degenitalized can be gratifying and this can increase sexual desire (Cardoso, 2006, Maia, 2011; Maior, 1988; Pinel, 1999).

From a neurological point of view, the autonomous nervous system is the main culprit for human excitement capacity and many psychological factors can prevent a person from feeling excitement by blocking their neurological signs. To define the excitement of the person with the spinal cord injury, it's necessary to know the level and extent of the injury and if the sacral reflex arc was affected. If the reflex pathway is maintained, which occurs in spinal cord injuries above the sacral segments, the reflex erection is possible, but in complete lesions, the psychogenic erection would already be inexistent. Men with complete upper lesions can maintain their reflex erection capacity, but not the psychogenic; in incomplete upper lesions, reflex erections would be normal and the psychogenic could exist. In the complete lower lesions, the reflex erections would be impossible and psychogenics would be possible and in incomplete lower lesions, both erections would be possible. However, in every case, the organic alterations depend on the emotional and social alterations (Cardoso, 2006; Maia, 2011, Maior, 1988; Pinel, 1999).

The orgasm, however, can be felt in some cases even though it's a complex phenomenon. Although the penile and vaginal sensations might not be felt in people who have spinal cord injuries, other physiological changes related to the orgasm, extragenital, for example, can be observed and felt by those people: other erogenous zones let the subject experience sensations of pleasure and corporal satisfaction or even the satisfaction of being with the other person. As a result of ejaculatory problems, masculine infertility is also frequent, mainly in complete lower lesions (Cardoso, 2006; Maior, 1988; Pinel, 1999).

In women, the ability to get pregnant is preserved, but changes in the sexual response can also occur, such as alterations in the clitoral or anal stimulation sensitivity, reduced lubrication and congestion of external genitalia. For men and women, orgasms are experienced more frequently in incomplete lesions or even the so-called "phantom orgasms" or "paraorgasms" that are pleasurable sensations after stimulation of the erogenous zones that are not affected by the lesion (Maia, 2006; Maior, 1988; Pinel, 1999; Salimene, 1995). Pinel (1999) explains:

"Sexual response involves profound changes in the body as a whole and not just non-genital: blood pressure and heart beat increases, the person becomes breatheless, with skin blushes. As well as the orgasms are not identical in intensity to the same person, the organic alterations will cause changes in the perception. [...]. Today we know that orgasm is possible after a spinal cord injury. Although it is not easy or automatic, orgasm can be built, regardless of erection, ejaculation or vaginal lubrication. This, however, usually involves a work of re-identification and redefinition of sensations [...]. The relearning of the spinal cord injured person goes further than physiotherapy and caring of bladder and intestines. It includes social, emotional and sexual restructuring that enables the person to life again" (Pinel, p.220).

Feminine reproduction is preserved after the lesion. In the case of men, the chance of ejaculation is low and some fertility treatments that can be used or recommended are: insemination, in vitro fertilization, gamete intrafallopian transfer, and intracytoplasmic sperm injection (Full-Riede, Hausmann & Schneider 2003) or electroejaculation, penile vibratory stimulation, pharmacological agents that induce ejaculation (Baer, 2003).

It's common for people with spinal cord injuries to make comparisons with their sex life before the injury, associate erections and orgasms as indispensable phenomenona of sexual intercourse and this increases feelings of failure, a higher degree of anxiety and depression that end up decreasing desire and excitement (Baer, 2003; Cardoso, 2006; Pinel, 1999). In addition, some authors (Ferri & Gregg, 1998; Silva & Albertini, 2007; Soares, Moreira & Monteiro, 2008) argue that socially determined gender questions influence coping with the disability in a different way. That is, the impact of acquired disability may have different psychosocial implications when it comes to men or women.

1.3.3 The sexuality counseling

The spinal cord injury also involves important psychological changes that must be considered in clinical treatments for this population. It is common, given the situation of extreme physical and emotional dependence of other people, spinal cord injured people express attitudes of rejection and denial of reality. There are also feelings of denial, grief, anger, and also reactions of depression and low self-esteem (Maior, 1988; Maia, 2006; Puhlmann, 2000).

"The most common psychological reactions of people who become physically disabled involve emotional dependence, rejection of reality attitudes, , alternated phases of depression and euphoria, loss of self-esteem, lack of confidence and satisfaction withown body, presence of inferiority and neglect feelings, decreased sexual desire, or excessive preoccupation with sexuality. There are also conflicts with body image and feelings of shame, fear and isolation appear, with concerns of social and sexual rejection"(Puhlmann, 2000, p.36).

In this sense, sexuality is an important issue that deserves special attention of professionals in rehabilitation programs, because sexual dysfunctions are common in people suffering from spinal cord injury. However, few health professionals have specific training to attend this demand (Major, 1988; Maia, 2011, Pinel, 1999).

The possibility of having a sexual dysfunction, especially among men is usually a humiliating and difficult condition because society in general values (and relates) social and sexual power. Sexual dysfunction treatment can be done with medication, always under the supervision of a doctor associated with sexual therapy or psychotherapy.

In the case of organic causes, the sexual dysfunctions are usually treated with the following treatments: intravenous, with the use of substances such as papaverine, phentolamine and prostaglandin E1 which basically is a penile injection that causes muscle tissue relaxation thus favoring the erection, b) urethral medication system with the introduction of prostaglandin E1 in the urethral canal c) oral medication such as sildenafil, which inhibits enzymes and assists smooth muscle with sexual stimulation. Other invasive treatments can be vascular surgery (low success rate) and even a penile implant, placed in the corpus cavernosum, which provides a mechanical or flexible hydraulic base. Other treatments can be no invasive and non-pharmacological, such as the use of a penis pump or penile rings (Baer, 2003; Ducharme & Gill, 1997; Full-Riede, Hausmann & Schneider 2003; Maior, 1988).

Problems such as urinary incontinence and spasticity are also common. Some techniques that decrease spasticity are recommendable like the appropriate temperature at the spot of sexual relation, massaging and antispasmodic medication. Also, there are certain positions that are important for stabilizing the articulation. In the case of incontinence, it's necessary that the bladder and rectum be emptied before the sexual relation and the use of mattress protectors and towels facilitate the necessary hygiene (Full-Riede, Hausmann & Schneider 2003).

Today, there are different tools for sexual dysfunction arising from spinal cord injuries spanning from sexual therapy technique that can help a person recover their sexual function response. Sexual therapy and rehabilitation process counseling for the population with physical disabilities, more specifically those with spinal cord injuries, have proven to be an important path to sexual health (Blackburn, 2002; Cardoso, 2006; Chigier, 1981; Maia, 2006; Maior, 1988; Puhlmann, 2000).

According to Maior (1988), sexual counseling programs for people with spinal cord injury are made from general strategies of sex therapy, including education and information, attitude change, elimination of anxiety before the performance, techniques of communication improvement and sexual behavior change, attending the impact of injury on sexual function. These programs should include an initial assessment phase, a work contract and planned counseling sessions that can be individual or in group.

At the initial assessment is necessary to survey the following information: (a) how was sexuality before and after the injury, (b) how is anal, bladder, urethra and genitalia sensitivity; if any drugs and medicines are used and how is the control of spasticity, (c) investigation of the sexual response: desire, arousal, orgasm, (d) investigation of the reproductive functions: menstruation, ovulation and ejaculation (Major, 1988; Maia, 2006). Maia (2006, p.182) says that is also necessary to investigate "sexual experiences prior to the injury, the frequency of interest and involvement in sexual activities, the most sensitive areas of the body, emotional relationships (whether or not a male or female partner) and desire to have children".

So, before intervention, a diagnostic evaluation is necessary in which information regarding sexual response before the injury is gathered, what the ideas about sexuality were, urinary function, intestinal and sexual evaluations are necessary, questions specifically related to masculinity and femininity. Objective data such as skin sensitivity, reflex or voluntary motor activity, the entirety of the reflex arcs, the level and degree of the spinal cord injury etc., are important for an appropriate diagnostic. The author adds that the more sexuality is seen as genital and focused on sexual functions, the more difficult sexual rehabilitation will be (Maior, 1988).

Some psychologists and sexual therapists have invested in specialized care for people with disabilities in order to ease possible dysfunctions arising from the disability, with several behavioral techniques or the use of equipment and "sex toys", such as vibrators and lubricants (Baer, 2003; Fürll-Riede, Hausmann & Schneider, 2003; Maior, 1988; Puhlmann, 2000).

"Sometimes people with disabilities need to be touched to have an erection. In this case, the accessories that stimulate the sensations of the skin across the body can be used. [...]. The stimulation of sexual organs can be produced with the caress and with the encouragement of sensory responses. To make this process dynamic, we can use contrast of cold and heat, or strength and weakness stimuli, seeking to provoke the activation of reflexes and deep sensation. The very touch of warm and cold hands can trigger reflex erection, massages with aromatic oils, or the subtle touch of soft tissues may facilitate arousal and are being widely used by disabled people. The so-called electric massagers and vibrators have facilitated not only male ejaculation in some cases of physical disability, where the ejaculatory reflex is impaired, but also the female orgasm, by strengthening local stimuli" (Puhlmann, 2000, p.105).

Along with this, it also takes time. Sexual readjustment does not happen immediately because restructuring conditions require time, trust and practice. Masturbation could be a form of practicing without any demands from the partner and help one get to know one's self sexually. It's necessary to have good communication, reduce anxiety and to clarify expectations, talking about feelings of pain under special conditions such as in spinal cord injury. It's necessary to relearn spontaneity, know how to express fantasies and sexual desires. Experimenting various sexual techniques such as oral and anal sex and trying different positions can be a very important resource for sexual rehabilitation (Baer, 2003; Ducharme & Gill, 1997; Kaufman, Silverg & Odette, 2003). Finally, feeling desired and having high self-esteem is essential for sexual rehabilitation (Baer, 2003).

Psychotherapy processes can help reconstruct the personal perception of what it's like to desire and be desirable, and this them should be given priority before applying sexual techniques. The first step for a subject is recognizing themselves as erotic human beings with disabilities. Other things should be considered along with the sexual response side: the existence of sensations of pain, fatigue, motor limitations, impaired ability to communicate assertively, unfavorable cognitive conditions (destructive thoughts and beliefs), privacy issues, difficulty in perceiving stimulation and finally, there can be issues due to side effects from medication. All of this needs to be considered. In any case, sexual health should be ensured, preventing the transmission of sexually transmitted diseases and unplanned pregnancy or situations of violence (Ducharme & Gill, 1997; Kaufman, Silverg & Odette, 2003).

In sexual rehabilitation, it's necessary to discuss the organically produced responses by the disability that in general, becomes problematic and join the psychological and social issues. The psychological issues are prioritized when attending people with disabilities beyond or together with sexual techniques, addressing subjects such as: body image, confronting myths and prejudice, restructuring of masculinity and femininity, reflecting about aesthetics standards, emotional difficulties that involve marital relationships, expectations about reproduction or even the difficulties of occurring sicknesses.

"From the point of view of attitudes, body image is a central issue. If a deficiency altered the appearance and/or mobility of a person beyond the accepted rules, the dislike of the body can assume proportions that interfere in the sexual encounter. Basically, if you hate the appearance of your body and how it behaves, will not be easy gladly offer it to a lover. Learn to love your own body, no matter how far he is from the ideal induced by the cinema (or even a more reasonable standard) takes time and is part of a wider process of self-acceptance"(Vash, 1988, p.90).

Fear of sexual dysfunction, feelings of inferiority, and problems with their companion or finding a sexual partner, lack of knowledge about how the body works, limitations due to spinal cord injuries, possibilities in sexual relations, possible problems and solutions are common self-esteem problems (Baer, 2003; Fürll-Riede, Hausmann & Schneider, 2003; Kaufman, Silverg & Odette, 2003; Maior, 1988; Puhlmann, 2000).

"A new image must be constructed from the reactions of this body and the reactions of others to a new body. [...]. Initially, many adopt an attitude of isolation and even of indifference to your problem. To establish their new body image, the spinal cord injured people need to know their limitations and modifications, including how to deal with equipment that use (wheelchair, crutches, urine collector), in a new experience of his own body; they must be able to expose this situation which is different to the others. [...]. People who base their self-esteem in physical capacity will probably struggle to readjust after injury [...]. Develop a new body image and restore self-esteem and sexual identity are the basic points for re-balancing of personality, appearing then confidence to assume a positive social and sexual role" (Major, 1988, p.25).

Finally, effective education programs and sexual rehabilitation should consider, above all, a few basic procedures.

In first place group work is required. Group sessions are indispensable for sharing experiences, frustrations and successes. Many subjects need to perceive that they are not alone in confronting sexual difficulties. Besides, family groups or couples are interesting alternatives to the extent that many times family support is necessary to recover self-esteem. Maior (1988, p.93) says that:

"It is agree that discussion groups should work from six to twelve people, including disabled people, partners and professionals. Although most programs work with groups, to each participant is given the option of complement individual counseling, individually or in couple with a partner"

Secondly, care should be given by a multidisciplinary team trained in the area, including psychologists, physical therapists, sexual therapists, doctors, etc. A treatment group that includes various professionals is essential in to whole care of people with a spinal cord injury (Baer, 2003; Cardoso, 2006; Maia, 2011; Major, 1988).

Sexual rehabilitation work should be comprehensive, considering emotional, labor issues, medical and disabling conditions, economic and social conditions, gender questions and sexual identity, ultimately other conditions need to be met by diverse professional if we hope to reach the person's overall sexual satisfaction.

2. Conclusion

Disability and sexuality are famous social phenomena, that's to say, they depend on social and historical representations about their conditions. Being disabled or dysfunctional manifests itself in the forms of personal and social normality that are socially constructed. Given these forms, feelings of maladjustment are common among people with and without disabilities. In the case of people with physical disabilities, these sentiments are common, because the disability is visible and stigmatizes the subject a deviant, which ends up being generalized for their sexuality.

The sexuality of people with physical disabilities reflects many social myths that were wrongfully put on these people such as having an atypical and unhappy sex life. However, despite possible organic difficulties, it's psychosocial questions that most reflect these difficulties, especially in the sexual area.

In this sense, the sexual rehabilitation of people with physical disabilities should include organized dysfunction treatment with the use of behavioral treatment and medication associated with sexual or psychotherapy that includes reflection on social models of normality, corporal difficulties, aesthetics and sexual function. It's important to consider manifestations such as problems with desire, excitement, orgasm or fertility, low self-esteem etc., result in internalized prejudice, in other words, the root is in the permanence of stigmatizing and prejudiced representations within society. We should join forces, ensuring teamwork (doctors, psychologists and other professional) and work the injured patients, family and/or spouse together.

3. Acknowledgment

Research Supported by FAPESP (Process No. 2011/07400-9) and publication supported by UNESP-Brazil (PROPe; PROINTER, Process No. 557-01 PDD-FUNDUNESP);

4. References

Amaral, L.A. (1995). *Conhecendo a deficiência:* em companhia de Hércules. São Paulo: Robe. (Série encontros com a psicologia).

Anderson, O. H. (2000). *Doing what comes naturally?* – dispelling myths and fallacies about sexuality and people with developmental disabilities. Illinois/ USA, High Tide Press.

Anderson, P.& Kitchin, R. (2000). Disability, space and sexuality: access to family planning services. *Social Science & Medicine, Oxford*, v. 51, n. 8, p. 1163-1173.

Aranha, M. S. F. (1995). Integração social do deficiente: análise conceitual e metodológica. *Temas em Psicologia*. São Paulo, n. 2, 63-70.

Baer, R. (2003). *Is Fred Dead?* - a manual on sexuality for men with spinal cord injuries. Pennsylvania: Dorrance Publishing.

Blackburn, M. (2002). *Sexuality & disability*. Oxford: Butterworth Heinemann.

Bozon, M. (2004). *Sociologia da Sexualidade*. (Maria de Lourdes Menezes, Trad.). Rio de Janeiro: Editora FGV.

Cardoso, J. (2006). *Sexualidade e Deficiência*. (Série Psicologia e Saúde). Coimbra/PT, Quarteto editora.

Chigier, E. (1981). Sexuality and disability: the international perspective. In: D. Bullard & S. Knight. *Sexuality & Physical Disability*: personal perspectives. (pp.134-142). Missouri/ USA, Mosby Company.

Daniels, S. (1981). Critical issues in sexuality and disability. In: D. Bullard & S. Knight (Orgs). *Sexuality & Physical Disability*: personal perspectives. (pp.5-17). Missouri/ USA, Mosby Company.

Ducharme, S.H. & Gill, K. M. (1997). *Sexuality after spinal cord injury- answers to your questions*. Baltimore, Maryland: Paul H. Brookes Publishing Co.

Edwards, M. L. (1997). Constructions of Physical disability in the ancient greek world- the community concept. In: D. T. Mitchell & S. L. Snyder (Eds.). *The Body and Physical Difference- discourses of disability*. (pp.35-50). Michigan, USA: University of Michigan.

Ferri, B. A.& Gregg, N. (1998). Women with disabilities: missing voices. *Women's Studies International Forum*, Oxford, v. 21, n. 4, 429-439.

Foucault, M. (1988). *História da sexualidade I* — a vontade de saber. (Maria Thereza Albuquerque, Trad.). Rio de Janeiro: Graal.

Foucault, M. (2002). *Os anormais*. (Eduardo Brandão, Trad.). São Paulo: Martins Fontes.

França, I.S.X. & Chaves, A.F. (2005). Sexualidade e paraplegia: o dito, o explícito e o oculto. *Revista Acta Paul. Enfermagem,18(3)*, 253-259.

Fróes, M. A. V. (2000). Sexualidade e deficiência. *Temas Sobre Desenvolvimento*, São Paulo, v. 8, n. 48, 24-29.

Fürll-Riede, C.; Hausmann, R. & Schneider, W. (2003). *Reabilitação Sexual do Deficiente*. (Raimundo Rodrigues Santos, Trad.). Rio de Janeiro: Revinter.

Giami, A. (2004). *O anjo e a fera: sexualidade, deficiência mental, instituição*. (Lydia Macedo, Trad.). São Paulo/SP, Casa do Psicólogo.

Goffman, E. (1988). *Estigma: notas sobre a manipulação da identidade deteriorada*. (Márcia Bandeira de Mello Leite Nunes, Trad.). 4. ed. Rio de Janeiro: Guanabara Koogan.

Kaufman, M.; Silverberg, C. & Odette, F. (2003). *The ultimate guide to sex and disability* – for all of us who live with disabilities, chronic pain e illness. (2a ed). Califórnia/USA, Cleis Press.

Loureiro, S. C. C.; Faro, A.C. M., & Chaves, E. C. (1997). Qualidade de vida sob a ótica de pessoas que apresentam lesão medular. *Revista Esc. Enf. USP, 31*(3): 347-367.

Maia, A.C.B (2006). *Sexualidade e Deficiências*. São Paulo/SP, Editora Unesp.

Maia, A. C. B. (2009). Sexualidade, Deficiência e Gênero: reflexões sobre padrões definidores de normalidade. In: R.D. Junqueira (Org.). *Diversidade Sexual na Educação: problematizações sobre homofobia nas escolas*. (Coleção Educação para todos). (pp.265-292). Brasília: Ministério da Educação, SECAD, UNESCO.

Maia, A.C.B. (2010). Conceito amplo de Sexualidade no processo de Educação Sexual. *Revista Psicopedagogia On Line*, 1-10.

Maia, A. C. B. (2011). *Inclusão e sexualidade na voz de pessoas com deficiências físicas*. Curitiba: Ed. Juruá.

Maia, A.C.B.; & Ribeiro, P. R.M. (2010). Desfazendo mitos para minimizar o preconceito sobre a sexualidade de pessoas com deficiências. *Revista Brasileira de Educação Especial, 16*(2): 159-176.

Maior, I. M. M. L. (1988). *Reabilitação sexual do paraplégico e tetraplégico*. São Paulo: Revinter.

Marques, C. A. (1997). Integração: uma via de mão dupla na cultura e na sociedade. In: M.T.E. Mantoan (Org.) *A integração de pessoas com deficiência:* contribuições para uma reflexão sobre o tema. (pp.18-23). São Paulo: Memnon.

Michell, D. T.& Snyder, S. L. (1997). Introduction- disability studies and the double bind of representation. (pp. 1-31). In: D.T. Mitchell & S. L. Snyder (Eds.). *The Body and Physical Difference- discourses of disability*. Michigan, USA: University of Michigan.

Omote, S. (1999). Deficiência: da diferença ao desvio. In: E. J. Manzini & P.R. Brancatti (Orgs.). *Educação especial e estigma:* corporeidade, sexualidade e expressão artística.(pp.3-21). Marília: Ed. UNESP.

Pinel, A. (1999). Educação sexual para pessoas portadoras de deficiências físicas e mentais. In: M. Ribeiro (Org.). *O prazer e o pensar:* orientação sexual para educadores e profissionais de saúde. (pp.211-226). São Paulo: Gente.

Pristley, M. (2001). *Disability and the life course*. New York: Cambridge.

Puhlmann, F.(2000). *A revolução sexual sobre rodas:* conquistando o afeto e a autonomia. São Paulo: O Nome da Rosa.

Ribas, J. B. C. (1998). *O que são as pessoas deficientes*. São Paulo: Brasiliense. (Coleção primeiros passos, v. 89).

Ross, P. R. (1998). Educação e trabalho: a conquista da diversidade ante as políticas neoliberais. In: L. Bianchetti & I. M. Freire (Orgs.). *Um olhar sobre a diferença:* interação, trabalho e cidadania. (pp.53-110). Campinas: Papirus. (Série educação especial).

Salimene, A. C. M. (1995). *Sexo:* caminho para a reabilitação: um estudo sobre a manifestação da sexualidade em homens paraplégicos. São Paulo: Cortez.

Siebers, T. (2008). *Disability Theory*. Michigan, USA: University of Michigan.

Silva, L.C. A. & Albertini, P. (2007). A re-invenção da sexualidade masculina na paraplegia adquirida. *Revista do Departamento de Psicologia UFF, v.19(1),* 37-48.

Soares, A.H.R., Moreira, M.C.N. & Monteiro, L.M.C. (2008). Jovens portadores de deficiência: sexualidade e estigma. *Revista Ciência & Saúde Coletiva, 13(1),* 185-194.

Soares, A.H.R., Moreira, M.C.N. & Monteiro, L.M.C. (2008). Jovens portadores de deficiência: sexualidade e estigma. *Revista Ciência & Saúde Coletiva, 13(1),* 185-194.

Sorrentino, A. M. (1990). *Handicap y rehabilitación-* uma brújula sistêmica en El universo relacional del niño com deficiências físicas. 1ª Ed. Barcelona, ES: Ediciones Paidós Ibérica.

Stoller, R. (1998). *Observando a Imaginação Erótica.* (Raul Fiker & Márcia Epstein Fiker, Trads.). Rio de Janeiro: Imago.

Tomasini, M. E. A. (1998). Expatriação social e a segregação institucional da diferença: reflexões. In: L. Bianchette & I. M. Freire (Orgs.). *Um olhar sobre a diferença:* interação, trabalho e cidadania. (pp. 111-134). Campinas: Papirus (Série educação especial).

Weeks, J. (1999). O Corpo e a sexualidade. In: G.L. Louro (1999). *O Corpo educado- pedagogias da sexualidade.* (Tomaz Tadeu da Silva, Trad.). (pp. 37-82). Belo Horizonte: Autêntica.

Werebe, M. J. G. (1984). Corpo e sexo: imagem corporal e identidade sexual. In: M. I. D'Avila Neto (Org.) *A negação da deficiência:* a instituição da diversidade. (pp.43-55). Rio de Janeiro: Achiamé/Socii.

Part 3

Animal Studies and Sexual Dysfunction

5

Paradigms for Preclinical Investigations of Female Sexual Function and Dysfunction (HSDD and FSAD)

Kelly A. Allers and Bernd Sommer
Boehringer Ingelheim Pharma GmbH & Co KG, Biberach an der Riss, Germany

1. Introduction

A prerequisite for successful discovery of treatment options for female sexual dysfunction is a deeper understanding of sexual function per se, e.g. which physiological systems are involved, and what goes wrong in a dysfunctional state.. The availability of animal models, which capture the physiological underpinnings of a disorder and have been shown to respond to existing clinical treatments are a major success factor in this endeavor. For example, the translational ability of penile erection models are extremely good, since they have high predictive value for drugs used to treat erectile dysfunction. Predictive validity of models of female sexual dysfunction is less well established. However, results from recent efforts to back-translate effects from drugs that have shown efficacy in clinical trials into laboratory animals provide promising starting points for a better disease understanding and model validation.

This chapter will briefly outline those models that have potential in helping understand female sexual function and dysfunction, followed by three examples (flibanserin, bremolantide, apomorphine) of how clinically efficacious compounds contributed to elucidate the physiology and pharmacology underlying both the natural and pathological states (Bechara et al. 2004; Caruso et al. 2004b; Clayton et al. 2010; Safarinejad 2008) of arousal and desire disorders, the major indications in terms of prevalence (Johannes et al. 2009).

Modeling a complex human behavior in the laboratory imparts many challenges. Only a few fundamental issues faced in the laboratory are similar in the clinic – ie. the necessity to define a 'normal' range of responses for a given function before attempting to assess a dysfunctional range. In the clinic, questionnaire based tools have been developed, that can define 'healthy' and 'dysfunctional' states of sexual behavior within human populations. Furthermore, the two behavioral domains 'desire' and 'arousal' become distinguishable when dysfunction is present (DeRogatis et al. 2011). This can principally be achieved in the lab too, since each species has a clear set of behaviors used to solicit sexual contact. Although it is not always easy to separate desire from arousal in rodents as these two components of the sexual response are temporally connected in a natural setting, they can be isolated and studied as distinct physiological pathways. However, in order to have translational relevance, such laboratory studies must address measures aligned with those used clinically. With this request a number of issues arise that are unique to working with laboratory animals and are eloquently summarized by a quote from Professor Jim Pfaus, a well respected researcher in sexual function. 'Animals don't lie, but they don't talk, either'. There is no equivalent of a Female Sexual Function Index (Rosen et al. 2000) or clinical interview for laboratory rats. The interpretation of their behavior is the responsibility of a well-informed researcher who is devoted to understanding the motivations and actions of the animals. At first sight physiological studies appear easier to translate, a neuron fires or it doesn't, a neurotransmitter is released or it isn't, and usually standard statistical methods scan determine if a given effect is significant. However, whether these data are meaningful to the human situation again requires a careful interpretation of the study.

The preclinical testing of a drug candidate would ideally occur in a 'disease' model, i.e. a model that mimics some or all of the symptoms observed in the human disorder. Since a drug to treat sexual dysfunction should be expected to restore natural sexual behavior, NOT to promote increased sexual behavior in a healthy individual, the appropriate model should show some hyposexuality. However, manipulations that induce a state of hyposexuality in animals are not without disadvantage to research. On one hand, these models will allow the investigator to assess a drug's ability to restore natural behavior. On the other hand, whatever hormonal/pharmacological/behavioral manipulation that was used to induce hyposexuality becomes a confound that may bias the experiment. Careful interpretation of the data is required, and preferably a known predictive ability for clinical efficacy within the model can provide confidence in its usefulness.

With the abovementioned clinically efficacious compounds, substantial multidisciplinary investigation has ensued to elucidate the pharmacological mechanism of action of these drugs. This is just the boost that female sexual dysfunction research has needed, clinically efficacious drugs that can be used in back-translation to validate animal models, and the resources of the pharmaceutical industry to tenaciously investigate pharmacological mechanisms.

2. Measuring 'desire' in animal models

There is no single definition of desire. The DSM-IV-R defines the primary symptom of Hypoactive Sexual Desire Disorder as 'Deficient or absent sexual fantasies and desire for sexual activity'(American Psychiatric Association 2000), which suggests that sexual desire is the presence of fantasies and the desire for sexual activity....although this is clearly not a functional working definition. Perhaps Agmo's strategy in his recent review - to simply consult the dictionary - is more relevant (Agmo et al. 2004). The Merriam Webster dictionary suggests desire is: **1:** conscious impulse toward something that promises enjoyment or satisfaction in its attainment, **2***a*: longing, craving *b* **:** sexual urge or appetite, **3:** a usually formal request or petition for some action (http://www.merriam-webster.com/dictionary). With this definition paradigms that assess the different components can be obtained. We can assess whether an animal is motivated to seek a partner for sexual activity and whether this activity was enjoyed using paradigms that allow the female rat to choose place, and timing of copulation (and sometimes the partner as well), and studies that determine if there was reward value to the encounter. Studies such as the bilevel pacing chamber, in which the female rat solicits the male with species specific behaviors demonstrate a type of 'request' for action. Craving can be assessed in a similar way as it has been done in studies of drug addiction and craving, by determining with operant tasks whether an animal will 'work' toward achieving a goal (sexual activity or drug of addiction).

There is a long history in the behavioral psychology literature regarding assessment of motivation, incentives, and reward in the study of sexual function and the interpretation of this data (Agmo et al. 2004; Matthews et al. 1997; Pfaus 1996; Pfaus 2009b). This literature is ultimately relevant to the study of sexual function and interpretation of the studies described herein, but it is beyond the scope of this chapter. What will follow is a short description of current models with potential use in studying both normal and pathological sexual behaviors, what kind of information they provide, and their utility in development of treatments for sexual desire dysfunction.

2.1 Behavioral models assessing sexual motivation

Behavioral models which are used to assess sexual motivation in general fall under two categories: those that measure directly the appetitive or proceptive behaviors used by females to show interest in a partner, and those that measure the reward value of a sexual encounter, providing a measure of the incentive to engage in sexual activity.

2.1.1 Behavioral models assessing appetitive/proceptive behaviors

Pacing chambers: Pacing chambers are experimental boxes designed to allow a female rodent the ability to 'pace' the amount of contact she has with the male. The bi-level chamber is a commonly used design. In this design, the chamber itself consists of two levels with ramps at either end, allowing the female to escape or pursue her partner over both levels (Mendelson et al. 1987; Pfaus et al. 1992). Another type of pacing chamber consists of a plexiglass cage with a barrier in the middle. The barrier contains an opening big enough for the female to pass through, but not the male; alternatively another type of escape route is provided such as a chamber adjacent to a testing arena (Paredes et al. 1999; Peirce et al. 1961). In both of these designs, the female can approach or avoid the male according to her own level of motivation. In these studies behaviors that are meant to 'solicit' the attention of the male (eg ear wiggles, hops and darts, etc.) can be readily measured. In addition, the response to male mounting attempts can be assessed. Pacing chambers are crucial to assessing motivation for sexual contact in a female rodent, as a paradigm that does not allow the female to control the pacing of sexual contact does not induce reward, and therefore decreases motivation (Paredes et al. 1997).

Partner Preference: Partner preference paradigms determine whether the test animal has more attraction to one animal over another. For example, a study examined whether a sexually receptive female rat prefers to spend time investigating another female rat, or a male rat (Clark et al. 2004). The goal of this type of study can be to determine what factors influence motivation for sexual contact as compared to social contact. In another study, female rats were allowed either paced copulation with almond-scented male rats or non-paced copulations with non-scented males. When entered into a partner preference study, the females solicited almond-scented males more than non-scented, suggesting the animals associated the scent with more rewarding sexual contact (Coria-Avila et al. 2005). Clearly there are many variations on partner preference studies that can be utilised, answering different questions related to motivated sexual behavior.

Primate models: Primate sexual behavior models provide an advantage over rodent models in that long-term primate pairs can be studied - mimicing the human situation. The hormone-dependency of primate sexual behavior is less strict than in rodents - again more like humans. Rhesus monkeys have commonly been used to assess proceptive behaviors.

However, primate models also introduce further complexities of social relationships and status, different social structures which can regulate sexual activity. In rhesus monkeys, it is well established that the laboratory setting can substantially alter 'normal' sexual motivation when these relationships cannot be controlled for (Wallen 1990). Marmosets are small primates that form long term pair-bonds and have been successfully utilised for studies of sexual motivation in a laboratory setting. This design has allowed detailed study of hormonal influences and pharmacological manipulations to be assessed for their effects on sexual behavior within the pair (Barnett et al. 2006; Kendrick et al. 1985).

2.1.2 Behavioral models assessing reward value of sexual activity

Place Preference: Place preference is a test in which an animal has a choice between two chambers, and learns to associate one with a rewarding experience (Tzschentke 2007). For example, at the beginning of an experiment, the animal is placed into a cage which is separated in half by a plexiglass divider, but with an opening through which the animal can pass freely. With no conditioned stimulus, the animal will have no preference between the two sides and spends equal time in both. However if an animal is taught to associate a positive experience in one chamber, then the animal will choose to spend time in the chamber in which the positive experience occurred. Alternatively, animals show a preference for a given chamber at the start of the test, and the experimental manipulation is used to change the preference to the alternate chamber. This test has been used to demonstrate a rewarding experience for paced sexual contact (Paredes et al. 1997).

Operant behavior designs: In operant behavior studies, the animal is taught that a sequence of behaviors will lead to a given outcome. For example, a female rat learns that pressing a lever will lead to access to a sexually active male rat (Bermant et al. 1966). In this situation, if the female rat is motivated to engage in sexual behavior, pressing the lever and achieving this access to a male serves as a reinforcer. In one such study, the male was removed following a mount, an intromission, or an ejaculation. The latency for the female to press the level for further contact was recorded. The response latencies were shortest when the females were only mounted, intermediate when intromissions occurred, and longest following ejaculation. These data indicate that the animal was more motivated to continue sexual contact before the male ejaculated than after (Bermant 1961).

2.2 Disorders of desire and potential animal models

Hypoactive sexual desire disorder (HSDD) is defined by the Diagnostic and Statistical Manual of Mental Disorders, Fourth Edition, Text Revision (DSM-IV-TR) as persistent or recurrent deficiency or absence of sexual fantasies and thoughts, and/or desire for, or receptivity to, sexual activity, which causes personal distress or interpersonal difficulties and is not caused by a medical condition or drug (American Psychiatric Association 2000). This disorder has a prevalence of between 6-10% in females assessed from the US population (Johannes et al. 2009; Simon 2010).

In designing preclinical experiments to investigate the biology of HSDD, the ideal would be a population of animals which actually exhibit the symptoms of this disorder with the same underlying neuropathology as patients. Clearly that is not possible. We can measure sexual motivation with the multiple behavioral models mentioned above, and in some situations distress and interpersonal difficulties may even be inferred from animal behavior such as aggressive rejection in rodents or fighting between primate pair-mates, there is no objective means of assessing thoughts or fantasies in animals. Furthermore, the underlying neuropathology of HSDD is essentially unknown. However, neuroimaging studies indicate that there are clearly differences in brain activation patterns of women suffering from HSDD when compared to healthy volunteers, confirming a neurological basis for symptoms (Arnow, 2009). With the substantial literature from preclinical studies, we are beginning to understand how the neurotransmitter pathways involved in sexual motivation not only function, but also how they can be dysfunctional. Michael Perleman introduced the concept of the 'Sexual Tipping Point'®, which incorporates the myriad of influences on a person when calculating their sexual desire (Perelman 2009). This concept describes the 'excitatory' and 'inhibitory' factors that are imparted by physiological, psychosocial, and cultural influences. Certainly from a neurobiological perspective, this concept holds true (Bancroft et al. 2009). Scientific evidence for this kind of balance in the neurobiology of desire has recently been reviewed, and an evidence based hypothesis generated for the underlying pathology of HSDD (Bancroft et al. 2009; Pfaus 2009b). Neurotransmitters such as dopamine and norepinephrine have a role in stimulating sexual activity, while serotonin plays an inhibitory role. Steroid and stress hormones also play a role in inducing sexual excitation or inhibition. These neurochemical pathways provide the 'balance' which can be tipped towards or away from motivation for sexual contact depending on intrinsic and environmental factors. The basic hypothesis for the neuropathology of HSDD is that either the systems regulating sexual excitation are inefficient, or the systems regulating inhibition are overactive, or both.

Preclinical studies have demonstrated multiple means of making a female animal 'hyposexual' by manipulating the excitatory and inhibitory pathways regulating sexual function. Following are descriptions and suggestions of what might be useful in drug development, for testing of potential compounds to treat HSDD.

Hormone manipulations: The simplest method of achieving low desire in animals is to remove hormone cycling by ovariectomy. Without further manipulation, rodents do not engage in sexual contact and this could potentially be used to assess compounds meant to restore sexual health (Lopez et al. 2007). However, ovariectomised animals are not an ideal model for HSDD since a large proportion of patients are premenopausal and do not show altered hormone status. They may, however, serve to model decreased libido in post-menopausal women. A further option is to exploit a rat's intrinsic hormone cycling. As a female rat moves from estrus into metestrus her physiology adapts by sending a 'stop' signal in the brain. This is hormonally mediated, but with correlated neurophysiological changes (Hawcock et al. 2010; Lopez et al. 2007; Richards et al. 2010). Attempting laboratory studies with only animals in metestrus is not easy, as this stage of their cycle lasts only a few hours, but subhormone priming can induce a steady-state that resembles metestrous behaviorally and in histopathology of vaginal smears (Hawcock et al. 2010). Furthermore, this type of priming has been used to show increases in sexual functioning with both apomorphine and melanotan II (the precursor to bremelanotide)(Allers et al. 2010d; Hawcock et al. 2010). In keeping with this idea, multiple studies using the behavioral paradigms mentioned above have been utilised with sub-estrus hormone primes which induce hyposexual behavior. Further investigation of the potential of sub-estrus hormone primes is certainly warranted.

Pharmacological manipulations: Two models have potential utility that use pharmacological alterations. First is SSRI-induced hyposexuality. Chronic or sub-chronic treatment with SSRIs in rats reduces sexual activity, although the effects on proceptivity compared to receptivity are unclear (Frye et al. 2010; Guptarak et al. 2010; Matuszczyk et al. 1998). While SSRI-induced sexual dysfunction would not be diagnosed as HSDD in humans, it is still a disorder which requires treatment, and it provides a model of hyposexuality in animals with a well characterised clinical correlate. A further model that was recently presented uses a disruption of early sexual reward which causes animals to 'learn' not to enjoy sexual contact. During her first sexual experiences a female rat is treated with naloxone, which diminishes the reward signal obtained. In further testing this results in a long lasting decrease in sexual contact (Pfaus et al. 2008).

Natural variation in sexual motivation: One study has demonstrated that within a normal population of female laboratory rats, a subgroup can be found which show more avoidance of sexual contact when presented with a male. Hence, when compared to the population as a whole, these animals are hyposexual. Translational relevance remains to be determined however, since apomorphine - a drug that has demonstrated clinical efficacy - does not induce increased sexual behavior in this model (Snoeren et al. 2011)

Marmoset model: A marmoset monkey model of hyposexual activity has been developed that utilises a combination of sub-optimal hormone priming and separation of the male and female pair mates to induce low levels of copulation on reunion. In addition, because the marmoset forms long-term pairs, a study design can include more than one hormone prime in a cross-over design to assess hormone dependence of compounds. This model has recently been used to assess the efficacy of flibanserin, a drug that has demonstrated efficacy in HSDD women in the clinic (Aubert et al. 2009; Tannenbaum et al. 2007).

3. Measuring arousal in animal models

There are two types of arousal that are relevant to sexual function, generalised arousal and peripheral arousal. Generalised arousal is a state of awareness or attention that is given to an organism's surroundings. An animal with a high state of generalised arousal has greater awareness of sensory cues, more motor activity, and a high degree of emotional reactivity. Peripheral arousal during sexual activity is the physiological preparation for sexual contact, such as vaginal and clitoral engorgement and lubrication.

Generalised arousal is relevant to sexual function as varying levels of sensory awareness or attention may be linked to motivation (Schober et al. 2011). In this sense, generalised arousal may be more closely linked to desire, than to peripheral arousal. Indications of decreased general arousal in sexual dysfunction, in particular women with HSDD support this link to desire. Women with HSDD show different brain activation patterns compared to healthy controls when viewing erotic videos, women with HSDD demonstrate differences in attending to sexual cues compared to healthy controls, and also have different electroencphalographic excitability as measured by the P300 wave when compared to both healthy controls and to women with arousal disorder (Arnow et al. 2009; McCall et al. 2006; Vardi et al. 2009). Consequently, it is possible that HSDD results from decreased generalised arousal or is a cause of it. Either way, it is clearly an important part of the sexual cycle. Generalised arousal is thought to be a key feature of an animal preparing to engage in any motivated behavior, not just sexual contact. If generalised arousal is necessary for motivated behavior, and motivated behavior is best measured in the aforementioned models, perhaps these behaviors are a good surrogate for generalised arousal.

Peripheral arousal related to sexual function typically refers to the autonomic response of the body as it prepares for sexual contact. In theory, the possibilities for preclinical research of the physiological mechanisms of arousal are endless. The circuitry from brainstem autonomic centers to the genitalia has been well studied, as have been the peripheral nerve innervation and structure and function of the genitalia. The understanding of healthy functioning arousal pathways, tissues, and biochemistry has grown substantially in recent years.

Below is a brief description of methods used to investigate peripheral arousal. Rather than review in detail the numerous techniques available, we will give a short description of the methods which can be utilised and the types of data generated.

3.1 Models of peripheral arousal

Lordosis behavior: It is arguable whether a lordosis reflex posture can be used as a measure of arousal. This is a posture adopted by female rats which allows the male access for intromission and ejaculation. The reason for including this here is twofold: female rats will exhibit lordosis even in non-paced mating situations where a 'rewarding' sexual experience does not occur and is therefore distinct from motivation or desire, and female rats will typically resist intromission if they are in a non-receptive hormone state or in pain. For these reasons, possibly lordosis may be a surrogate marker for arousal, in that physiologically, her body may be prepared for sexual contact and it is not uncomfortable to engage in copulation.

Vaginal blood flow models: Typically these types of studies are carried out in aneasthetised animals, usually rats or rabbits (Beharry et al. 2003; Giuliano et al. 2010; Hale et al. 2003). A basic paradigm uses peripheral nerve stimulation (ie pudendal or pelvic) to stimulate blood flow to the clitoris and vagina. These studies have been critical in elucidating the mechanisms by which blood flow to the genitals is regulated, and the neurotransmitters and hormones involved in such regulation. The blood flow itself can be measured by techniques, such as plethysmography or laser doppler flowmetry. In addition to the standard rate or amplitude of flow, further characterisation of blood flow as measured by laser doppler can elicit surrogate measures of autonomic activation to the vagina (Allers et al. 2010d; Allers et al. 2010c). These measures are obtained by fast Fourier transform analysis of the oscillations within blood flow and are similar to those used to assess heart rate variability. Using this type of analysis responses to naturally arousing stimuli (a male rat) and experimental manipulations meant to induce arousal (drugs, nerve section, hormone status) are observed.

In vitro studies: Studies on gential tissues also help to define the intricate biochemical and physiological mechanisms for healthy sexual functioning (Aughton et al. 2008; Wilson et al. 2009). These types of studies may investigate the mechanisms involved in vaginal smooth muscle contraction and relaxation, lubrication, or neurotransmitter release from innervating nerves. In addition, one unique model utilises an ex vivo brain tissue assay which shows responses that are highly predictive of lordosis behavior. In a drug development project where increased lordosis could be predictive of clinical efficacy, this assay provides an ideal tool for early drug screening (Booth et al. 2010).

3.2 Disorders of arousal and potential animal models

Female sexual arousal disorder (FSAD) is defined by the Diagnostic and Statistical Manual of Mental Disorders, Fourth Edition, Text Revision (DSM-IV-TR) as the inability to attain or maintain until completion of sexual activity adequate lubrication in response to sexual excitement (American Psychiatric Association 2000). Unfortunately, this definition does not truly seem to describe many FSAD patients since several studies have now shown that a patient will rate her subjective feelings of arousal quite low, but tends to show a normal genital response (Laan et al. 2008; Rellini et al. 2006). Classifying patients into subgroups of mainly genital arousal, or subjective arousal dysfunction in studies using VPA begins to show some differences, but subjective assessments remain the best diagnostic tools (Both et al. 2010; Salonia et al. 2010). In healthy women, there is not always agreement between subjective and physiologically measured responses either, perhaps due to interoceptive differences in attending to one's own genital physiology.

Even though there is a wealth of information on healthy arousal responses, there is no evidence based hypothesis for the neuropathology of FSAD. Clear differences in sympathetic responsiveness has been demonstrated in patients as compared to controls using procedures such as hyperventilation or extreme exercise (Brotto et al. 2009; Meston 2000). This points to a pathology in the systemic autonomic nervous system, or central-autonomic interface, rather than in the genitalia.

The majority of models above cannot provide translational disease models for FSAD, since vaginal vasocongestion is not affected in a large number of women with FSAD, and the likely pathology is within the circuitry of the autonomic or central nervous system. Only one technique above has demonstrated that it can actually distinguish between healthy controls and women with FSAD, and has been demonstrated to have predictive utility.

Slow oscillations in vaginal blood flow: In this model, laser Doppler flowmetry or vaginal plethysmograph can be used to record blood flow within the vaginal wall (Allers et al. 2010d; Allers et al. 2010c). Rather than assessing peak amplitudes, rate or other typical measures, the trace is analysed by fast Fourier transform (FFT) to elucidate the oscillatory charactistics of flow. This technique is well established in vascular research and these oscillations are known to reflect autonomic nervous system input to the tissue being studied. In this way, these measures are a surrogate of autonomic input. When measured in the vagina, the changes seen during sexual arousal paradigms are specific to the vagina, meaning they do not occur in other tissues simultaneously. This method has been used to differentiate human patients, correlates highly with subjective arousal in both healthy and FSAD women, and has been used in animals to show arousal inducing effects of apomorphine and melanotan II, in addition to natural arousal (exposure to sexually active male). Upon apomorphine administration animals in metestrus respond with increased slow oscillations in this model, at the same doses that induce restoration of sexual behavior in a partner-preference test (Hawcock et al. 2010). This model has not yet been used clinically to demonstrate restoration of natural arousal in FSAD women with a drug candidate, but has great potential as a translational model for investigation of drugs to treat FSAD.

4. Lessons from drug discovery

The process of drug discovery requires that a target (eg receptor, enzyme, etc.) be identified with a reasonable hypothesis for why it is engaged in a given disease state. This hypothesis is then rigorously tested within the laboratory with tool compounds and drug candidates. Alternatively, and typical of the sexual health field, a prosexual side effect is noticed for a given drug candidate, and this is quickly followed up to assess its potential for therapeutic use in sexual medicine. This process leads to a substantial amount of research into pathways, disease states, and pharmacological mechanisms regarding a particular target being generated. Within sexual health groups in the pharmaceutical industry recent targets have included dopamine receptors, serotonin receptors, and melanocortin receptors. The following examples demonstrate how the process of drug discovery and new drugs available for testing has contributed substantially to the scientific understanding of sexual function and dysfunction.

4.1 Apomorphine

Drug development teams have adopted multiple strategies for assessing dopamine receptors as a drug target, including assessing the roles of individual dopamine receptor subtypes, dopamine reuptake, or using a classical dopamine receptor agonist (apomorphine) in different formulations. Apomorphine is a non-selective dopamine agonist was first discovered in 1869 and over time has been used as an emetic, a treatment for alcohol and morphine addictions, and to improve symptoms of Parkinson's Disease (Subramony 2006).

Dopamine has long been known to be a modulator of sexual function. There are decades of literature reporting pro-sexual effects of dopamine agonists but also reports of the same paradigms producing reduced sexual behavior. Much research has focussed on elucidating the hormone dependence of effects, the regions of the brain where increased or decreased dopamine occurs during sexual contact in efforts to investigate the real role of dopamine in sexual function and where discrepancies in data may come from. Many review articles have highlighted ongoing questions related to dopamine in sexual function (Meisel et al. 2006; Paredes et al. 2004; Peeters et al. 2008; Pfaus 2009a; Stolzenberg et al. 2011b; Stolzenberg et al. 2011a).

Regardless of the scientific debates over how dopamine regulates sexual function, clinical evidence has indicated that stimulating dopamine receptors may provide help for women with sexual dysfunction (Bechara et al. 2004; Caruso et al. 2004a). For this reason, studies were undertaken to investigate further why apomorphine can have opposing effects on sexual behavior in rodents.

Using a partner preference paradigm in which a rat chooses to actively investigate either a sexually vigorous male or a castrated male, a measure of active investigation can be utilised to determine sexual interest compared to social interest. In this paradigm, female rats that are ovariectomised and given a sub-hormone prime to resemble metestrus do not show a preference for either male rat. Upon apomorphine treatment, a dose dependent increase in preference for the sexually vigorous male is observed. When this study is run with animals that have been fully hormonally primed to resemble behavioral estrous, they show a clear preference for the sexually vigorous male, which is decreased by apomorphine treatment (Hawcock et al. 2010). These data indicate that when ALL other conditions are equal dopamine receptor agonism can have the exact opposite effect simply by artificially placing the animal into different stages of the estrous cycle.

Further investigations suggest that the opposing effects of apomorphine occur in the naturally cycling animal in metestrus compared to estrous. Using the FFT analysis of laser doppler flowmetry in rats, these differential effects of apomorphine are also present. Metestrus animals had a significant increase in slow oscillatory activity of blood flow, which in this model is indicative of sexual arousal (Allers et al. 2010d). Furthermore, this increase could not be blocked by the peripheral antagonist domperidone, but could be attenuated with the centrally acting antagonist haloperidol, indicating apomorphine's actions did originate in the brain (Allers et al. 2010c). In estrous animals, apomorphine elicited a decrease in slow oscillatory activity indicating decreased arousal. The dose ranges in both

metestrus and estrous animals which had effects in this model are the same as those in the partner-preference model.
An electrophysiological study was undertaken to further understand the underlying mechanisms for the observed differences in apomorphine actions. Neurons from the paraventricular nucleus, a nucleus important for sexual function and hormonally regulated, were studied in animals from all four stages of the estrous cycle. Firing rates from this nucleus varied substantially across the estrous cycle, with metestrous rates being the highest. In addition subpopulations of neurons were identified: slow neurons which increase in response to apomorphine, and fast neurons which decrease in response to the drug. A greater proportion of the fast neurons were evident in metestrous, accounting for the higher mean firing rate, and leading to relatively greater decreases upon apomorphine (Richards et al. 2010).
Taken together, these data suggest that during metestrous, a neurological 'stop' signal has been physiologically delivered to the animal which is reflected the animal's behavioral disinterest in a sexual partner. This 'stop' signal is sensitive to, and can be reversed by apomorphine administration. This reversal manifests as increased interest in a sexual partner and increased sexual arousal. An underlying mechanism may be the inhibition of a fast-firing population of neurons within the paraventricular nucleus of the brain.

4.2 Bremelanotide

The peptide α-melanocyte stimulating hormone (MSH) is a product of the proopiomelanocortin pro-hormone. This peptide has long been known to be involved in regulation of energy homeostasis and has been suggested as a target for number medical indications (Hedlund 2004).
In the mid-1980s, a group at the University of Arizona synthesized two highly potent MSH analogues (Hadley et al. 1998). One compound, deemed Melanotan I (MTI) was licensed out and further characterised for utility as a tanning drug, given the known role of MSH in pigmentation. A further analogue, Melanotan II (MTII) was developed which was smaller and the hope was that this would aid in its absorption and tissue distribution. The investigator decided to assess for himself whether this second analogue had the tanning capability seen with MTI and proceeded to dose himself. While it is unclear whether he did achieve a tan, what the investigator reports was an "unrelenting" erection lasting 8 hours. Not long after, this compound was licensed out for further development as a sexual dysfunction treatment candidate. PT-141 is the active metabolite of MTII and ultimately became the drug development lead compound and was renamed bremelanotide.
Clincal trials in women have demonstrated that bremelanotide increases sexual desire and arousal in women with arousal disorders (Diamond et al. 2004; Diamond et al. 2006; Safarinejad 2008). In one study, using vaginal plethysmography to assess vasocongestion, even though subjective scores were increased over placebo, there was no change in vasocongestion measures as compared to controls, confirming that vaginal vasocongestion is not a suitable method for assessing efficacy of compounds (Diamond et al. 2006).
Prior to the discovery and development of bremelanotide, melanocortin receptors were not considered to be of great interest within the sexual medicine field. Since that time, a surge of interest has appeared, and along with it a boost in scientific research investigating the mechanisms involved.
Bremelanotide is an agonist at melanocortin 3 and 4 (MC3 and MC4) receptors, whose primary localisation is in the hypothalamic regions of the brain (Molinoff et al. 2003). The

most evidence currently points to action within either the medial pre-optic area (MPOA) or the paraventricular nuclues (PVN) or both. Behavioral studies in pacing chambers have demonstrated that peripheral administration of bremelanotide increases proceptive behaviors in female rats with different hormone primes. In addition, injection of the drug directly into the MPOA results in the same effect (Pfaus et al. 2007). In keeping with this data, peripheral injection of bremelanotide results in increased activation of MPOA neurons as measured by c-fos. In addition to bremelanotide's actions on proceptivity, the parent compound MTII has also been demonstrated to induce arousal in rats using the laser doppler method with FFT analysis of slow oscillatory activity (Allers et al. 2010d).
In male rats, a similar study demonstrates that following administration of bremelanotide c-fos activation occurs within the PVN of the hypothalamus (Molinoff et al. 2003). To assess if this is a potential pathway in females, further investigation was undertaken in naturally cycling estrus rats. Pseudorabies virus (PRV) injection to the clitoris and vagina resulted in transsynaptic labeling present in both the PVN and the MPOA. Furthermore, neurons that were double-labeled for PRV and the melanocortin 4 receptor were found in both the PVN and MPOA, indicating melanocortin pathways exist from both of these regions to the genitalia (Gelez et al. 2010). Between 4 and 8% of the PRV labeled neurons were triple-labeled for both the melanocortin 4 receptor and oxytocin. These data demonstrate direct pathways from both the PVN and the MPOA to the genitalia that could be part of bremelanotide's mechanism of action through activation of melanocortin 4 receptors on oxytocin neurons.

4.3 Flibanserin

Flibanserin was discovered in 1990 as part of a program investigating targets for depression (Borsini et al. 1997). This compound was developed based on a very sound rationale for why agonist activity at post-synaptic 5-HT1A receptors and antagonism of 5-HT2A receptors combined would be beneficial to patients with major depressive disorder (Borsini et al. 2002). Unfortuantely, during Phase II trials for depression, flibanserin was not superior to the positive control, paroxetine (Kennedy 2010).
Within the Phase II trials, patients were given the ASEX questionnaire to assess sexual function. Flibanserin treatment improved sexual function in 70% of the patients. Development of flibanserin for depression was discontinued but restarted development for the indication of hypoactive sexual desire disorder. Following several Phase III clinical trials with flibanserin in premenopausal women, the data indicating increased desire and decreased distress following chronic flibanserin treatment is substantial (Clayton et al. 2009; Goldfischer et al. 2009; Jolly et al. 2009).
Following the reassignment of this drug, the search for a mechanism of action began. Within sexual function research, 5-HT1A receptor agonism has long been known to reduce sexual behavior (Ahlenius et al. 1989; Mendelson et al. 1986; Uphouse et al. 1991). The finding that a 5-HT1A agonist is prosexual in women was puzzling. Treatment of rats in pacing chambers either at full estrous priming or sub-hormonal priming also indicated that rats increased proceptive behaviors with chronic flibanserin treatment, and hence, sexual motivation - eliminating the possibility of a species difference in 5-HT1A actions (Allers et al. 2010b; Greggain et al. 2010). Acute dosing of flibanserin has no effect on sexual behavior in rodents.
In pair-bonded marmosets, a study was conducted to compare the effects of chronic flibanserin treatment with that of a commonly used 5-HT1A agonist, 8-OH-DPAT. In this study, flibanserin induced increased affiliative behavior in both pair mates, although only

the females were treated. 8-OH-DPAT induced increased aggression between pairmates after treatment of females alone (Aubert et al. 2009). The result is that flibanserin is clearly not a typical 5-HT1A receptor agonist, but has unique properties that contribute to its mechanism of action.

A key to the difference in flibanserin pharmacology is it's ability to act only at post-synaptic 5-HT-1A receptors. A study by Marazziti et al. demonstrated that in human brain, flibanserin has low nanmolar potency at 5-HT1A receptors in the prefrontal cortex, but none at 10μM in the dorsal raphe nucleus (Marazziti et al. 2002). The 5-HT1A receptors in the dorsal raphe nucleus are responsible for regulating serotonin release throughout the brain and typical 5-HT1A agonists will inhibit this release. Post-synaptic receptors are located outside of the dorsal raphe nucleus and have many different functions, including regulating release of all monoamines. To determine how flibanserin administration affects monoamine release two microdialysis studies were undertaken. The first investigated acute dosing while measuring serotonin, dopamine, and norepinephrine in three regions of the brain: the prefrontal cortex, the dorsal raphe, and the hippocampus (Invernizzi et al. 2003). The surprising result was that flibanserin administration decreased serotonin in the prefrontal cortex and dorsal raphe, but not the hippocampus. Recent evidence suggests that hippocampal serotonin is regulated primarily by presynaptic 5-HT1A receptors within the dorsal raphe, so the interpretation for this study is that by acting only at post-synaptic receptors flibanserin can affect serotonin release in selected brain areas. The following microdialysis study indicated that dopamine and norepinephrine are also affected in regionally selective patterns upon chronic dosing (Allers et al. 2010a). Potentially the most significant finding was that within the prefrontal cortex, an area important for general arousal and motivation, basal levels of dopamine and norepinephrine were increased selectively in the prefrontal cortex out of the regions studied (prefrontal cortex, nucleus accumbens, hypothalamic medial preoptic area).

HSDD patients have been shown to have altered cortical reactivity and demonstrate differences in attending to sexual cues (McCall et al. 2006; Vardi et al. 2009). Flibanserin, by increasing two neurotransmitters known to be involved in sexual desire, selectively in regions responsible for attention and awareness, may act to restore these functions (Stahl et al. 2011).

5. Conclusions

In conclusion, the development of centrally acting clinically efficacious drugs (albeit none yet with FDA approval) to treat sexual dysfunction, and the development of new models for assessing drug effects preclinically has given the sexual sexual function research field a much needed boost. New models of dysfunction can now be validated as they are developed and translation to human dysfunction can be better established.

6. References

Agmo, A., Turi, A. L., Ellingsen, E., and Kaspersen, H.2004Preclinical models of sexual desire: conceptual and behavioral analysesPharmacol.Biochem.Behav.783379404

Ahlenius, S., Larsson, K., and Fernandez-Guasti, A.1989Evidence for the involvement of central 5-HT1A receptors in the mediation of lordosis behavior in the female ratPsychopharmacology (Berl).984440444

Allers, K. A., Dremencov, E., Ceci, A., Flik, G., Ferger, B., Cremers, T. I., Ittrich, C., and Sommer, B.2010aAcute and repeated flibanserin administration in female rats modulates monoamines differentially across brain areas: a microdialysis studyJ.Sex Med.7517571767

Allers, K. A., Gelez, H., Sommer, B., and Giuliano, F.2010bEffects of flibanserin on appetitive and consummatory aspects of sexual behavior in ovariectomized female rats primed with estrogen and progesteroneSociety for Neuroscience Meeting Abstracts595

Allers, K. A., Richards, N., Scott, L., Sweatman, C., Cheung, J., Reynolds, D., Casey, J. H., and Wayman, C.2010cII. Slow oscillations in vaginal blood flow: regulation of vaginal blood flow patterns in rat by central and autonomic mechanismsJ.Sex Med.7310881103

Allers, K. A., Richards, N., Sultana, S., Sudworth, M., Dawkins, T., Hawcock, A. B., Buchanon, T., Casey, J. H., and Wayman, C.2010dI. Slow oscillations in vaginal blood flow: alterations during sexual arousal in rodents and humansJ.Sex Med.7310741087

American Psychiatric Association2000Diagnostic and Statistical Manual of Mental Disorders, 4th edition, text revision.

Arnow, B. A., Millheiser, L., Garrett, A., Lake, Polan M., Glover, G. H., Hill, K. R., Lightbody, A., Watson, C., Banner, L., Smart, T., Buchanan, T., and Desmond, J. E.1-23-2009Women with hypoactive sexual desire disorder compared to normal females: A functional magnetic resonance imaging studyNeuroscience.1582484502

Aubert, Y., converse, A., Sommer, B., Allers, K. A., and Abbott, D. H.2009Comparison of flibanserin with the 5-HT1A agonist (+)-8-OH-DPAT in affecting interactions between male-female marmoset pairsJ.Sex Med.6(suppl 5)422

Aughton, K. L., Hamilton-Smith, K., Gupta, J., Morton, J. S., Wayman, C. P., and Jackson, V. M.2008Pharmacological profiling of neuropeptides on rabbit vaginal wall and vaginal artery smooth muscle in vitroBr.J.Pharmacol.1552236243

Bancroft, J., Graham, C. A., Janssen, E., and Sanders, S. A.2009The dual control model: current status and future directionsJ.Sex Res.462-3121142

Barnett, D. K., Bunnell, T. M., Millar, R. P., and Abbott, D. H.2006Gonadotropin-releasing hormone II stimulates female sexual behavior in marmoset monkeys Endocrinology. 1471615623

Bechara, A., Bertolino, M. V., Casabe, A., and Fredotovich, N.2004A double-blind randomized placebo control study comparing the objective and subjective changes in female sexual response using sublingual apomorphineJ Sex Med12

Beharry, R. K., Hale, T. M., Wilson, E. A., Heaton, J. P., and Adams, M. A.2003Evidence for centrally initiated genital vasocongestive engorgement in the female rat: findings from a new model of female sexual arousal responseInt.J.Impot.Res.152122128

Bermant, G.6-2-1961Response Latencies of Female Rats during Sexual Intercourse Science. 133346617711773

Bermant, G. and Westbrook, W. H.1966Peripheral factors in the regulation of sexual contact by female ratsJ.Comp Physiol Psychol.612244250

Booth, C., Wayman, C. P., and Jackson, V. M.2010An ex vivo multi-electrode approach to evaluate endogenous hormones and receptor subtype pharmacology on evoked and spontaneous neuronal activity within the ventromedial hypothalamus; translation from female receptivityJ.Sex Med.7724112423

Borsini, F., Cesana, R., Kelly, J., Leonard, B. E., McNamara, M., Richards, J., and Seiden, L.1997BIMT 17: a putative antidepressant with a fast onset of action? Psychopharmacology (Berl). 1344378386

Borsini, F., Evans, K., Jason, K., Rohde, F., Alexander, B., and Pollentier, S. 2002 Pharmacology of flibanserin CNS. Drug Rev. 82117142

Both, S., Laan, E., and Schultz, W. W.2010Disorders in sexual desire and sexual arousal in women, a 2010 state of the artJ.Psychosom.Obstet.Gynaecol.314207218

Brotto, L. A., Klein, C., and Gorzalka, B. B.2009Laboratory-induced hyperventilation differentiates female sexual arousal disorder subtypes Arch. Sex Behav. 384463475

Caruso, S., Agnello, C., Intelisano, G., Farina, M., Di Mari, L., and Cianci, A.2004aPlacebo-controlled study on efficacy and safety of daily apomorphine SL intake in premenopausal women affected by hypoactive sexual desire disorder and sexual arousal disorder Urology 635

Caruso, S., Agnello, C., Intelisano, G., Farina, M., Di, Mari L., and Cianci, A.2004bPlacebo-controlled study on efficacy and safety of daily apomorphine SL intake in premenopausal women affected by hypoactive sexual desire disorder and sexual arousal disorder Urology. 635955959

Clark, A. S., Kelton, M. C., Guarraci, F. A., and Clyons, E. Q.2004Hormonal status and test condition, but not sexual experience, modulate partner preference in female ratsHorm.Behav. 455314323

Clayton, A., jayne, C., Jacobs, M., Kimura, T., Pyke, R., and Lewis-D'Agostino, D.2009Efficacy of flibanserin as a potential treatment for hypoactive sexual desire disorder in North American premenopausal women: Results from the DAHLIA trial. J Sex Med 6 (suppl 5) 408

Clayton, A. H., Dennerstein, L., Pyke, R., and Sand, M.2010Flibanserin: a potential treatment for Hypoactive Sexual Desire Disorder in premenopausal womenWomens Health (Lond Engl.).65639653

Coria-Avila, G. A., Ouimet, A. J., Pacheco, P., Manzo, J., and Pfaus, J. G.2005Olfactory conditioned partner preference in the female ratBehav.Neurosci.11937167250735-7044

DeRogatis, L. R., Clayton, A. H., Rosen, R. C., Sand, M., and Pyke, R. E.2011Should sexual desire and arousal disorders in women be merged?Arch.Sex Behav.402217219

Diamond, L. E., Earle, D. C., Heiman, J. R., Rosen, R. C., Perelman, M. A., and Harning, R.2006An effect on the subjective sexual response in premenopausal women with sexual arousal disorder by bremelanotide (PT-141), a melanocortin receptor agonistJ.Sex Med.346286381743-6095

Diamond, L. E., Earle, D. C., Rosen, R. C., Willett, M. S., and Molinoff, P. B.2004Double-blind, placebo-controlled evaluation of the safety, pharmacokinetic properties and pharmacodynamic effects of intranasal PT-141, a melanocortin receptor agonist, in healthy males and patients with mild-to-moderate erectile dysfunction Int. J. Impot. Res. 1615159

Frye, C. A. and Rhodes, M. E.2010Fluoxetine-Induced Decrements in Sexual Responses of Female Rats and Hamsters Are Reversed by 3alpha,5alpha-THPJ.Sex Med.

Gelez, H., Poirier, S., Facchinetti, P., Allers, K. A., Wayman, C., Alexandre, L., and Giuliano, F.2010Neuroanatomical evidence for a role of central melanocortin-4 receptors and oxytocin in the efferent control of the rodent clitoris and vaginaJ.Sex Med.7620562067

Giuliano, F., Pfaus, J., Srilatha, B., Hedlund, P., Hisasue, S., Marson, L., and Wallen, K.2010Experimental models for the study of female and male sexual functionJ.Sex Med.7929702995

Goldfischer, E. R., Breaux, J., Katz, M., Kaufman, J., Smith, W. B., Patel, P., Mikl, J., Sand, M., and Pyke, R.2009Efficacy of continued flibanserin treatment in premenopausal women with hypoactive sexual desire disorder: Results from the ROSE study.J Sex Med20096(suppl 5)114

Greggain, J., Allers, K. A., Sommer, B., and Pfaus, J.2010Effects of repeated flibanserin treatment on appetitive sexual behaviors in male and female ratsJ Sex Med7(suppl 6)395

Guptarak, J., Sarkar, J., Hiegel, C., and Uphouse, L.2010Role of 5-HT(1A) receptors in fluoxetine-induced lordosis inhibitionHorm.Behav.582290296

Hadley, M. E., Hruby, V. J., Blanchard, J., Dorr, R. T., Levine, N., Dawson, B. V., al-Obeidi, F., and Sawyer, T. K.1998Discovery and development of novel melanogenic drugs. Melanotan-I and -IIPharm.Biotechnol.11:575-95.575595

Hale, T. M., Heaton, J. P., and Adams, M. A.2003A framework for the present and future development of experimental models of female sexual dysfunction Int. J. Impot. Res. 15 Suppl 5:S75-9.S75S79

Hawcock, A. B., Dawkins, T. E., and Reynolds, D. S.2010Assessment of 'active investigation' as a potential measure of female sexual incentive motivation in a preclinical non-contact rodent model: observations with apomorphine Pharmacol. Biochem. Behav. 952179186

Hedlund, P.2004PT-141 PalatinCurr.Opin.Investig.Drugs.54456462

Invernizzi, R. W., Sacchetti, G., Parini, S., Acconcia, S., and Samanin, R.2003Flibanserin, a potential antidepressant drug, lowers 5-HT and raises dopamine and noradrenaline in the rat prefrontal cortex dialysate: role of 5-HT(1A) receptorsBr.J.Pharmacol.139712811288

Johannes, C. B., Clayton, A. H., Odom, D. M., Rosen, R. C., Russo, P. A., Shifren, J. L., and Monz, B. U.2009Distressing sexual problems in United States women revisited: prevalence after accounting for depressionJ.Clin.Psychiatry.701216981706

Jolly, E., Clayton, A., Thorp, J., Kimura, T, Sand, M., and Pyke, R.2009Efficacy of flibanserin 100 mg qhs as a potential treatment for hypoactive sexual desire disorder in North American premenopausal womenJ Sex Med6(Supp 5)465

Kendrick, K. M. and Dixson, A. F.1985Effects of oestradiol 17B, progesterone and testosterone upon proceptivity and receptivity in ovariectomized common marmosets (Callithrix jacchus)Physiol Behav.341123128

Kennedy, S.2010Flibanserin: initial evidence of efficacy on sexual dysfunction, in patients with major depressive disorderJ.Sex Med.71034493459

Laan, E., van Driel, E. M., and van Lunsen, R. H.2008Genital responsiveness in healthy women with and without sexual arousal disorderJ.Sex Med.5614241435

Lopez, H. H., Wurzel, G., and Ragen, B.2007The effect of acute bupropion on sexual motivation and behavior in the female ratPharmacol.Biochem.Behav.873369379

Marazziti, D., Palego, L., Giromella, A., Mazzoni, M. R., Borsini, F., Mayer, N., Naccarato, A. G., Lucacchini, A., and Cassano, G. B.2002Region-dependent effects of flibanserin and buspirone on adenylyl cyclase activity in the human brain Int. J. Neuropsychopharmacol.52131140

Matthews, T. J., Grigore, M., Tang, L., Doat, M., Kow, L. M., and Pfaff, D. W.1997Sexual reinforcement in the female ratJ.Exp.Anal.Behav.683399410

Matuszczyk, J. V., Larsson, K., and Eriksson, E.1998Subchronic administration of fluoxetine impairs estrous behavior in intact female rats Neuropsychopharmacology. 196492498

McCall, K. and Meston, C.2006Cues resulting in desire for sexual activity in womenJ.Sex Med.35838852

Meisel, R. L. and Mullins, A. J.12-18-2006Sexual experience in female rodents: cellular mechanisms and functional consequencesBrain Res.112615665

Mendelson, S. D. and Gorzalka, B. B.19865-HT1A receptors: differential involvement in female and male sexual behavior in the ratPhysiol Behav.372345351

Mendelson, S. D. and Gorzalka, B. B.1987An improved chamber for the observation and analysis of the sexual behavior of the female ratPhysiol Behav.3916771

Meston, C. M.2000Sympathetic nervous system activity and female sexual arousal Am. J. Cardiol. 862A30F34F

Molinoff, P. B., Shadiack, A. M., Earle, D., Diamond, L. E., and Quon, C. Y.2003PT-141: a melanocortin agonist for the treatment of sexual dysfunction Ann. N.Y. Acad.Sci.994:96-102.96102

Paredes, R. G. and Agmo, A.2004Has dopamine a physiological role in the control of sexual behavior? A critical review of the evidence Prog.Neurobiol.733179226

Paredes, R. G. and Alonso, A.1997Sexual behavior regulated (paced) by the female induces conditioned place preferenceBehav. Neurosci.1111123128

Paredes, R. G. and Vazquez, B.11-1-1999What do female rats like about sex? Paced matingBehav.Brain Res.1051117127

Peeters, M. and Giuliano, F.2008Central neurophysiology and dopaminergic control of ejaculationNeurosci.Biobehav. Rev.323438453

PEIRCE, J. T. and NUTTALL, R. L.1961Self-paced sexual behavior in the female ratJ.Comp Physiol Psychol.54:310-3.310313

Perelman, M. A.2009The sexual tipping point: a mind/body model for sexual medicineJ.Sex Med.63629632

Pfaus, J., Giuliano, F., and Gelez, H.2007Bremelanotide: an overview of preclinical CNS effects on female sexual functionJ.Sex Med.4 Suppl 42692791743-6095

Pfaus, J. G.1996Frank A. Beach award. Homologies of animal and human sexual behaviorsHorm.Behav.3031872000018-506X

Pfaus, J. G.2009bPathways of sexual desireJ.Sex Med.6615061533

Pfaus, J. G.2009aPathways of sexual desireJ.Sex Med.6615061533

Pfaus, J. G. and Pfaff, D. W.1992Mu-, delta-, and kappa-opioid receptor agonists selectively modulate sexual behaviors in the female rat: differential dependence on progesteroneHorm.Behav.264457473

Pfaus, J. G., serrano, S, and Coria-Avila, G.2008Blockade of optiod receptors during early sexual experience decreases sexual desire in female ratsSociety for Neuroscience Meeting Abstracts97.15

Rellini, A. and Meston, C.2006The sensitivity of event logs, self-administered questionnaires and photoplethysmography to detect treatment-induced changes in female sexual arousal disorder (FSAD) diagnosisJ.Sex Med.32283291

Richards, N., Wayman, C., and Allers, K. A.2010Neuronal activity in the hypothalamic paraventricular nucleus varies across the estrous cycle in anesthetized female rats: effects of dopamine receptor agonismJ.Sex Med.7311041115

Rosen, R., Brown, C., Heiman, J., Leiblum, S., Meston, C., Shabsigh, R., Ferguson, D., and D'Agostino, R., Jr.2000The Female Sexual Function Index (FSFI): a multidimensional self-report instrument for the assessment of female sexual functionJ.Sex Marital Ther.262191208

Safarinejad, M. R.2008Evaluation of the safety and efficacy of bremelanotide, a melanocortin receptor agonist, in female subjects with arousal disorder: a double-blind placebo-controlled, fixed dose, randomized studyJ.Sex Med.54887897

Salonia, A., Giraldi, A., Chivers, M. L., Georgiadis, J. R., Levin, R., Maravilla, K. R., and McCarthy, M. M.5-11-2010Physiology of Women's Sexual Function: Basic Knowledge and New FindingsJ.Sex Med.

Schober, J., Weil, Z., and Pfaff, D.2011How generalized CNS arousal strengthens sexual arousal (and vice versa)Horm.Behav.595689695

Simon, J. A.2010Low sexual desire--is it all in her head? Pathophysiology, diagnosis, and treatment of hypoactive sexual desire disorderPostgrad.Med.1226128136

Snoeren, E. M., Chan, J. S., de Jong, T. R., Waldinger, M. D., Olivier, B., and Oosting, R. S.2011A new female rat animal model for hypoactive sexual desire disorder; behavioral and pharmacological evidenceJ.Sex Med.814456

Stahl, S. M., Sommer, B., and Allers, K. A.2011Multifunctional pharmacology of flibanserin: possible mechanism of therapeutic action in hypoactive sexual desire disorderJ.Sex Med.811527

Stolzenberg, D. S. and Numan, M.2011bHypothalamic interaction with the mesolimbic DA system in the control of the maternal and sexual behaviors in ratsNeurosci.Biobehav.Rev.353826847

Stolzenberg, D. S. and Numan, M.2011aHypothalamic interaction with the mesolimbic DA system in the control of the maternal and sexual behaviors in ratsNeurosci.Biobehav.Rev.353826847

Subramony, J. A.2006Apomorphine in dopaminergic therapyMol.Pharm.34380385

Tannenbaum, P. L., Schultz-Darken, N. J., Woller, M. J., and Abbott, D. H.2007Gonadotrophin-releasing hormone (GnRH) release in marmosets II: pulsatile release of GnRH and pituitary gonadotrophin in adult females J. Neuroendocrinol. 195354363

Tzschentke, T. M.2007Measuring reward with the conditioned place preference (CPP) paradigm: update of the last decadeAddict.Biol.123-4227462

Uphouse, L., Montanez, S., Richards-Hill, R., Caldarola-Pastuszka, M., and Droge, M.1991Effects of the 5-HT1A agonist, 8-OH-DPAT, on sexual behaviors of the proestrous rat Pharmacol. Biochem. Behav. 393635640

Vardi, Y., Sprecher, E., Gruenwald, I., Yarnitsky, D., Gartman, I., and Granovsky, Y.2009The p300 event-related potential technique for libido assessment in women with hypoactive sexual desire disorder J. Sex Med. 6616881695

Wallen, K.1990Desire and ability: hormones and the regulation of female sexual behaviorNeurosci.Biobehav.Rev.1422332410149-7634

Wilson, L. A., Wayman, C. P., and Jackson, V. M.2009Neuropeptide modulation of a lumbar spinal reflex: potential implications for female sexual functionJ.Sex Med.64947957

6

Development of Male Sexual Function After Prenatal Modulation of Cholinergic System

Alekber Bairamov[1], Alina Babenko[1], Galina Yukina[2], Elena Grineva[1], Boris Komikov[2], Petr Shabanov[3] and Nikolay Sapronov[3]
[1]*Almazov Federal Heart, Blood and Endocrinology Centre, St. Petersburg,*
[2]*Saint Petersburg State Medical Academy named after I. I. Mechnikov,*
[3]*Institute Experimental Medicine,*
Nord-West Division of the Russian Academy of Medical Science, St. Petersburg,
Russia

1. Introduction

Embryonal period of ontogenesis plays an important role in the brain development which is defined, first of all, by genetical factors. Normal flow of the process can be disturbed also under the influence of many environmental factors which affect, both a differentiation of neurones, and on a neurotransmitter choice in them used for communications with the proximate cells (Le Douarin, 1981; Pendleton, 1998). The majority of the factors attacking developing brain during this period, break a normal ontogenesis of neurotransmitter systems: NA, 5-HT, DA and ACh that shows high sensitivity of a brain in critical periods of the development (Williams, 1992; Oliff, 1999; Qiao, 2004).

A variety of neurochemical changes in the embryonic brain, induced by exposure to neurotropic compounds during the prenatal period, result in the development of functional impairments and behavioral disorders in the adult offspring. The mechanisms of action of many chemical factors on the developing fetal brain during early ontogenesis are in most cases mediated by alterations in the formation and functioning of brain neurotransmitter systems, including the cholinergic system, whose CNS function is associated with memory, learning, and behavioral processes (Yamada et al., 1986; Buzsaki, 1989; Everitt & Robbins, 1998; Levin & Slotkin, 1988; Zoli et al., 1999). During the period of neuron development, actions on cholinergic mechanisms lead to delays in cell differentiation which correlate with cognitive and behavioral deficits in fertile offspring (Yamada et al., 1986; Levin & Simon, 1998; Beer et al., 2005).

Prenatal exposure to neurotoxins (nicotine, organochlorine compounds, barbiturates), which have cholinotropic properties, produces long-lasting changes in neurotransmitter functions in early ontogenesis with the subsequent development of neurobehavioral anomalies and affective disorders in pubescent individuals (Seidler et al., 1992; Barinaga, 1996; Slotkin, 2004). Thus, embryonic exposure to nicotine leads to alterations to cell proliferation and differentiation, resulting in long-term changes to synaptic function (Peters, 1986; Lichtensteiger, 1988). Binding to N-cholinergic receptors in catecholamine-containing neurons in the fetal brain, nicotine disrupts the expression of these transmitters

(Lichtensteiger et al., 1988; Dani & Heinemann, 1996). Prenatal exposure to nicotine predominantly damages cholinergic, noradrennergic, and dopaminergic projections in the brain during postnatal life, with later cognitive and behavioral dysfunction in adult offspring (Naeye & Peters, 1984; Milberger et al., 1996; Fergusson et al., 1998; Orlebeke et al., 1997; Weissman et al., 1999; Slotkin et al., 2001).

The neurobehavioral teratogenic actions of barbiturates are also mediated by disrupted functioning of septohippocampal cholinergic conducting pathways, which is accompanied by a deficiency of synaptic transmission and accompanying hippocampus-related behavioral deficit (Wallace, 1984; Smith et al, 1986; Yanai, 1984, 1996; Steingart et al,, 2000; Azmitia, 2001; Beer et al. 2005; Beer et al., 2005). Phenobarbital, previously used for the prophylaxis of neonatal hyperbilirubinemia and bleeding in neonatal children, is a teratogenic factor in relation to behavior in both humans and animals (Yanai, 1984; Wallace, 1984; Smith et al, 1986). Experimental exposure to organochlorine compounds, like other neurotoxins with cholinotropic properties, damages cholinergic conducting pathways and leads to long-term alterations to the cholinergic system (Lauder, 1985; Dreyfus, 1998; Qiao et al., 2002; Slotkin et al., 2002; Slotkin, 2004). Dysfunction of cholinergic neurons plays a significant role in behavioral disorders seen in adult rats given organochlorine compounds during the prenatal period (Sherman et al., 1981).

Behavioral abnormalities as long-term consequences of prenatal exposure to various factors are generally difficult to observe because of the large phenotypic variability of the developing organism (Nicholls, 2000). There is great value in studying sexual behavior in these situations, as sexual functions are the most sensitive and susceptible aspects of reproduction in males and, as has been demonstrated, are regulated by the activities of several neurotransmitter systems, including the cholinergic (Bitran & Hull, 1987; Mas et al., 1987; Hull et al., 1988; Retana et al., 1993; Gladkova, 2000).

In addition, despite many studies of substances with cholinotropic properties and adverse influences on the developing brain during the prenatal period, the literature lacks reports of the behavioral effects of prenatally administered selective cholinolytics.

Taking into consideration all these statements, the purpose of the present research is study of known selective blockers of M- and N-cholinergic systems, prescribed in various terms of a prenatal period, on development dynamics of neurotransmitter systems of the rats embryos brain, and track their dynamics in an adolescent period and in adulthood in comparison to the behavioural sexual status in the paste for a sexual behavior at rats males.

Tasks of the present part of work were the following:

- Research of sexual abnormalities of the 3-4-month-old rats males and possibility of their pharmacological correction.
- Analysis of the effects of selective M- and N-cholinergic systems blockers prenatal influence on dynamics of neurotransmitter systems development of 20-day-old rats embryos brain, in various terms of a gestation.
- Study of the neurochemical status of brain structures, participating in formation and regulation of neuroendocrinal and behavioural function of 2-month-old rats that were effected by prenatal influence M- and N-cholinolytics.

2. Methods

Investigations were performed on Wistar rats from the Rappolovo supplier, Russian Academy of Medical Sciences (Leningradskaya Oblast). Several series of experiments were performed. Female rats with a known date of pregnancy were obtained by mating females in proestrus-estrus with males. The day on which sperm were seen in vaginal smears was taken as the first day of pregnancy. Pregnant females, at different stages of gestation (9–11, 12–14, and 17–19 days of pregnancy), were given three i.m. injections (once daily) of the N-cholinoblocker ganglerone (10 mg/kg), while other groups received injections of the M-cholinoblocker methylbenactyzine (2 mg/kg) at the same time points. Doses were determined on the basis of the selectivities of cholinolytic actions and the absence of nonspecific actions. Control groups of females received injections of physiological saline. Experiments offspring groups (12–14 individuals per group) were formed in accord with the timing of prenatal administration of ganglerone (groups G10, G13, and G18, respectively) and methylbenactyzine (groups M10, M13, and M18). The offspring of intact rats served as the control group.

Behavioral studies were performed on rat offspring aged 3.5–4 months. Sexual experience was acquired in four sequential tests with receptive females. Sexual activity parameters were assessed using a standard sexual behavior test (3). Adult rats were kept in individual cages with food and water available *ad libitum*, in a room with controlled temperature and under an inverted 12 × 12 h light cycle (light off at 09:00 h). Tests for sexual behavior were done during the dark phase of the cycle and under dim red light illumination The test male was placed in the study chamber, of size 40 x 40 x 30 cm, for 5 min prior to presentation of a sexually susceptible female. Experiments were performed in dim red illumination. Receptivity in sterilized females was induced by sequential administration of estradiol dipropionate (25 mg, 48 h before the experiment) and progesterone (500 g, 4 h before the experiment). Components of sexual activity were recorded visually for 15 min in tests 1 and 4. The numbers of components of sexual behavior (mountings, intromissions, and ejaculations) and their latent periods were registered. During each behavioral test, the behavioral components recorded were mount latency (time from the introduction of a receptive female to the first mount), intromission latency (time from the introduction of a receptive female to the first intromission), ejaculation latency (interval between the first intromission and ejaculation), and postejaculatory interval (interval between the first ejaculation and the next intromission).

Neurochemical studies were performed using brains from 20-day embryos and brain structures (hypothalamus, hippocampus) from rat offspring two month age. The concentrations of the neurotransmitters dopamine (DA), noradrenaline (NA), and serotonin (5-HT) in brain tissues were measured by high-performance liquid chromatography using a Beckman System Gold with an LC-4C electrochemical detector. Brain structures were extracted on a cryostat at -20°C and were stored in liquid nitrogen until chromatographic analysis. Peaks were separated on a SphereClone 5 μ ODS 2 chromatography column (250 × 4.60 mm) with a Phenomenex precolumn. The mobile phase consisted of citratephosphate buffer pH 3.5, acetonitrile (88 ml/liter), and octanesulfonic acid (43 mg/liter). Chromatographic peaks were identified and assessed quantitatively in relation to peaks obtained from internal standards.

Serum hormone levels were assayed by immunoenzyme analysis using standard biochemical kits (Chema, Access) on a Uniplan immunoenzyme analyzer. Statistical analysis. Results were compared with control data and analyzed statistically by analysis of variance (ANOVA) on Origin 7.0.

3. Sexual function of 3,5-4-month-old males offsprings subjected to prenatal exposure of selective M- and N-cholinoblockers

For the purpose of revealing sexual function abnormalities of puberal offsprings of male rats their primary sexual activity and dynamics of acquisition of sexual experience has been investigated. Offsprings of intact rats were control group.

The results obtained from behavioral studies showed that administration of methylbenactyzine and ganglerone to pregnant females at different periods of gestation induced long-term impairments to sexual function in pubescent offspring. In the first test, there were significant reductions in sexual function on appearance of primary sexual activity in offspring subjected to prenatal exposure to ganglerone (groups G10–G18) (Fig. 1). The males of this group included the large proportion of individuals in which all elements of sexual behavior were absent (henceforth - "inactive" individuals). The proportion of inactive males among the offspring of groups M10–M18 was significantly smaller and, after acquisition of sexual experience, decreased to 1–2 individuals in terms of both copulative (Fig. 1, B) and ejaculatory (Fig. 1, A) functions.

As not all males demonstrated sexual activity including the final component of sexual behavior, i.e., ejaculation, a group of males showing incomplete copulatory activity (mounting and intromission, without ejaculation) was identified (Fig. 1, B).

Analysis of the elements of sexual behavior over time (from test 1 to test 4) showed that the most marked differences in the intensity of acquiring sexual experience between offspring in groups G10–G18 and M10–M18 were seen in relation to the final element of copulation, i.e., ejaculatory activity. Offspring of groups G10–G18 showed positive dynamics only for copulatory activity, while there were no changes in the amounts of ejaculatory activity with the increase in sexual experience. The proportions of inactive males in terms of this parameters in groups G10–G18 amounted to about half of the total number of animals (from four to seven individuals) used for testing sexual behavior (Fig. 1).

Changes in the time parameters of sexual functions during four sessions of sexual behavior showed a similar dynamic for copulatory components. As sexual experience was acquired, the latent periods of the main elements of sexual behavior decreased, to a greater extent in males of groups M10–M18 than in offspring of groups G10–G18, and were comparable with control values (for example, mounting latencies are shown in Fig. 2).

Thus, more males which were inactive in the sexual behavior test (both before and after acquisition of sexual experience) were seen among the offspring of groups G10–G18 (particularly in males of group G10). A characteristic feature of the sexual behavior of males in these groups was the absence of marked dynamics of the acquisition of sexual experience by the fourth test.

Studies of the structure of sexual behavior in males with acquired sexual experience showed that sexual function in males of groups G10–G18 was characterized by very low values for the copulatory components of sexual behavior, with long latent periods. Levels of ejaculatory activity were extremely low (0.40 ± 0.16 ejaculations among the G10 offspring compared with 1.90 ± 0.18 in the control group).

The long latency of mounting in males of group G10 and, to a lesser extent, group G13, provides evidence of a significant alteration in the motivational component of sexual behavior (Fig. 2). In males of groups M10–M18 with acquired sexual experience, differences in sexual activity as compared with control offspring were less marked, with the exception of group M10, in which there was a significantly lower value of the ejaculatory component, without any change in the latent period of mounting. Analysis of the effects of prenatal administration of substances at different periods of pregnancy showed that sexual function in the offspring was most sensitive to injection of the N-cholinolytic ganglerone at 9–11 and 12–14 days of gestation and the M-cholinolytic methylbenactyzine at 9–11 days of gestation. The comparative analysis of the other parametres of males sexual behaviour from the groups G10-G18 and M10-M18 with the acquired sexual experience showed more appreciable sexual dysfunctions of offsprings G10-G18 in comparison with the offsprings, that were subjected to prenatal influence of methylbenactyzine (tab. 1). The structure of sexual function of males from group G10-G18 with the acquired sexual experience was characterized by very low value of copulatory components and their high latence. Level of ejaculatory activity of all groups G10-G18 was extremely low and authentically differed from control group.

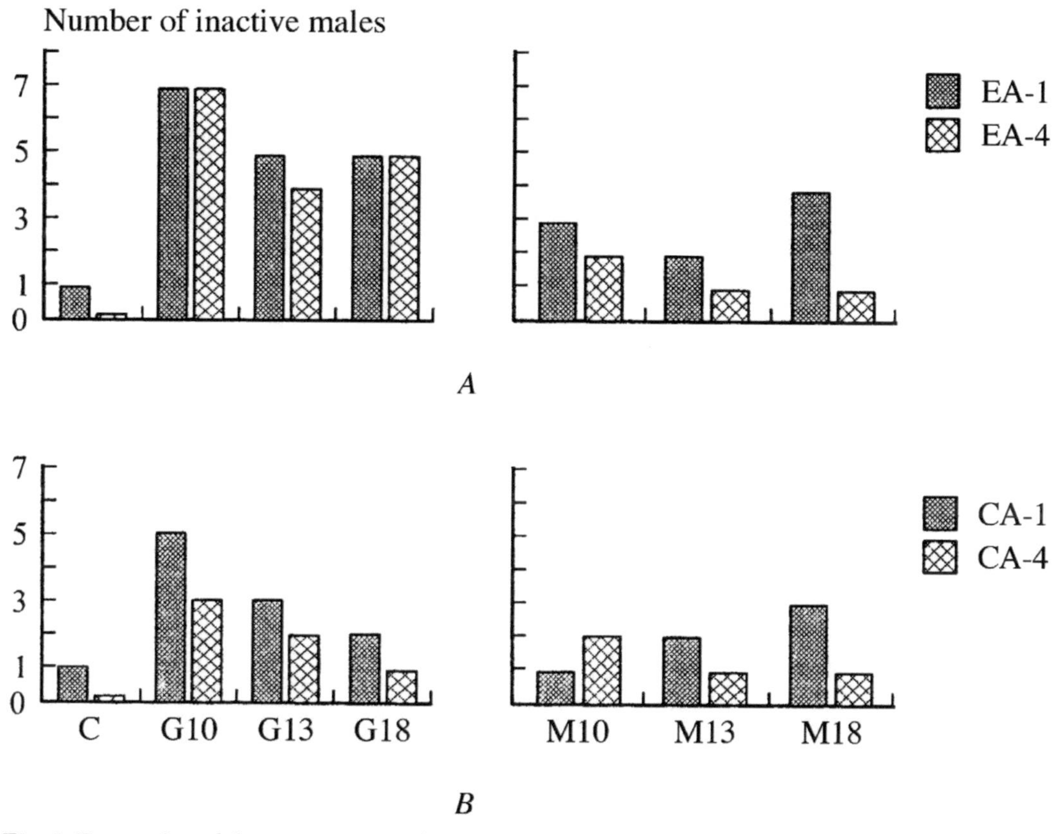

Fig. 1. Dynamics of the acquisition of sexual activity in offspring; data based on ejaculatory and copulatory (mountings and intromissions) behavior in four sequential tests for sexual behavior (data from tests 1 and 4) (n = 14). Dark columns show numbers of inactive males in the first test; shaded columns show inactive males in the fourth test. **A)** Number of inactive males in terms of ejaculatory activity (EA) in offspring subjected to prenatal exposure to ganglerone at 9–11, 12–14, and 17–19 days of pregnancy (groups G10, G13, and G18, respectively) or methylbenactyzine (groups M10, M13, and M18, respectively) compared with control offspring; **B)** number of inactive males in terms of incomplete copulatory activity (CA) (mountings and intromissions) in offspring of these groups.

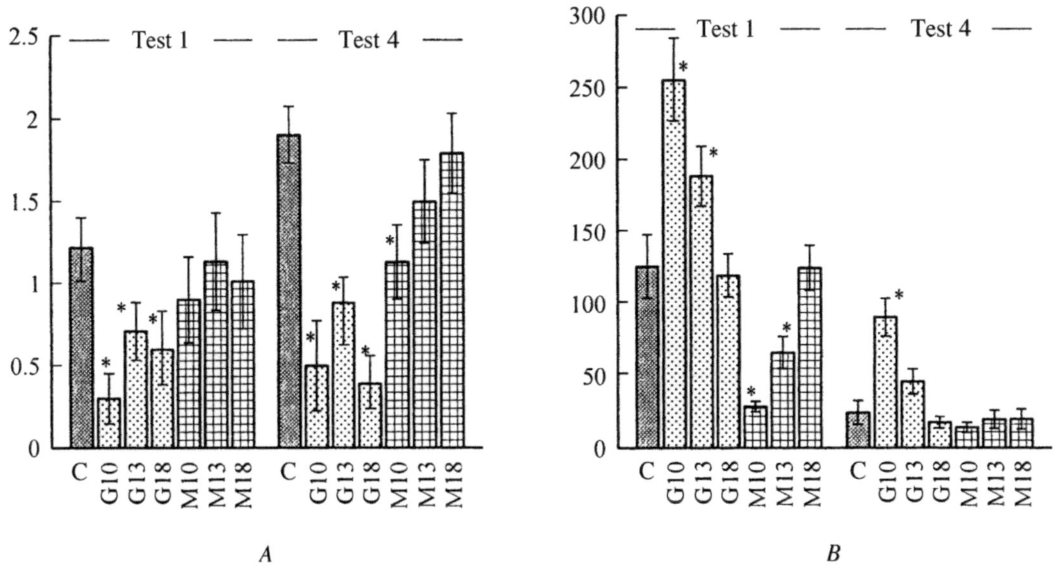

Fig. 2. Parameters of sexual behavior in the offspring of rats subjected to prenatal exposure to methylbenactyzine (M) or ganglerone (G) in the first and fourth tests. A) Latent period of mating. The ordinate shows time, sec; B) number of ejaculations throughout the sexual behavior test period. *p < 0.05 compared with the control group. For further details see caption to Fig. 1.

Thus, the results of the present study show that treatment of pregnant females with ganglerone (and, to a lesser extent, methylbenactyzine) at different periods of pregnancy leads to behavioral abnormalities in the offspring: there were significant reductions in sexual function and the intensity of the acquisition of sexual experience.

The studies of Gladkova (1994) showed that the intensity of sexual behavior in males depends on having the appropriate experience. As a rule, sexual activity in the first test with receptive females was low, but increased from test to test such that the quantitative levels of sexuality in male rats were essentially constant after the third contact with females. Administration of the N-cholinolytic to pregnant females at 9–11 and 12–14 days of gestation facilitated the appearance of significantly larger proportions of inactive males among their offspring, these animals being characterized by an extremely low dynamic of the acquisition of sexual experience as compared with control offspring. In these males (groups G10–G13), acquisition of sexual experience was followed by sexual functions with significant disruption of ejaculatory activity and the central motivational element of sexual behavior. These data indicate that ganglerone modulation of the N-cholinergic system in the developing fetal brain leads to changes in the quantitative and qualitative characteristics of elements of sexual behavior in pubescent offspring.

In groups with prenatal exposure to the M-cholinolytic, changes in sexual function were noted only in offspring of group M10 - which had a significantly reduced level of the ejaculatory component as compared with control offspring, though this was not linked with changes in the motivational aspect of sexual behavior. These data showed that prenatal changes in the activity of the M-cholinergic system lead to insignificant behavioral consequences in pubescent offspring. Thus, the results obtained here provide evidence that prenatal alterations to the N-cholinergic and, to a lesser extent, the M-cholinergic system induce long-term sexual impairments in the pubescent offspring.

Groups	Mounts (n)	latency of mount (sec)	Intromissions (n)	latency of intromission (sec)	Ejaculation (n)	latency of ejaculation (sec)	Interejaculatory interval (sec)	Restoration period (sec)
Control_1	9,70 ±1,93	123,2±42,8	6,10±1,08	166,2±42,6	1,20±0,20	369,8±65,0	504,0±49,5	328,0±26,7
Control_4	15,8±2,15	23,6±28,3	9,50±1,65	73,8±35,8	1,90±0,18	297,4±48,9	362,6±39,5	270,3±15,6
G-10_1	6,8±2,70	255,6±149,3	3,90±1,80	320,8±139,3	0,30±0,15	449,0±44,2	-	288±39,7
G-10_4	9,80±3,22*	89,1±33,6*	6,10±2,09*	50,7±25,5	0,50±0,27*	312,7±49,8	457,5±56,5	325,3±29,0
G-13_1	17,6±3,11	188,8±60,4	9,40±1,36	237,9±54,7	0,70±0,21	521,3±85,6	509,0±0,00	282,5±11,8
G-13_4	17,1±3,1	26,0±9,0	11,4±2,1	53,9±16,0	0,90±0,17*	278,8±53,0	403,5±29,1	307,7±23,2
G-18_1	12,5±2,54	117,5±34,1	5,20±1,17	201,5±43,7	0,60±0,22	288,4±30,4	562,0±34,5	327,2±17,8
G-18_4	28,9±3,76*	16,9±3,30*	15,2±2,19*	69,1±15,3	1,07±0,16*	525,8±22,2*	-	348,8±26,9
M-10_1	18,3±3,57	27,8±3,44	11,0±2,0	58,5±10,2	0,89±0,26	512,7±88,1	509,5±49,5	328,2±44,4
M-10_4	17,8±3,90	13,4±4,97*	10,0±2,31	46,1±9,72	1,13±0,23*	571,6±88,4*	479,5±36,5*	296,3±36,2
M-13_1	13,6±3,54	64,7±17,5	7,50±1,95	91,3±16,9	1,13±0,30	310,5±44,4	461,0±55,2	336,3±38,4
M-13_4	12,3±2,16	19,3±3,98	5,000,96*	69,7±5,66	1,50±0,27*	227,7±36,4	453,8±21,4*	345,6±20,8
M-18_1	6,70±1,84	123,0±26,6	4,00±1,23	165,2±33,2	1,00±0,30	223,3±29,5	428,0±45,8	318,7±33,6
M-18_4	13,9±4,2	18,4±3,62	6,8±1,83*	53,8±5,48	1,8±0,25	252,4±56,5	436,5±30,2	278,2±19,6

*-p < 0.05 compared with the control group.
Abbr : **n**- number; **sec**- second of time.

Table 1. Parameters of sexual behavior in the mature male rats subjected to prenatal exposure to ganglerone (G) or methylbenactyzine (M) at different periods of prenatal development compared with the control group. (M±m).

We believe that sexual dysfunction in adult offspring induced by prenatal exposure to cholinolytics is due to changes to neuronal and endocrine mechanisms. The mechanisms regulating sexual behavior are known to be mediated to a significant extent by neuronal structures located in the preoptic zone of the hypothalamus and to be activated by different neurotransmitter systems, including the cholinergic system (Dorner, 1989). Cholinergic activation of the preoptic area via M1 muscarinic receptors is critical for normal coitus (Hull et al., 1988a; Hull et al., 1988b; Retana et al., 1993). The absence of long-term sexual dysfunction in offspring subjected to prenatal exposure to methylbenactyzine provides evidence that impairments to sexual function in males are not mediated by the M-cholinergic system of the brain.

4. Neurochemical subsequences of prenatal exposure of selective M- and N-cholinoblockers in the rat fetus brain on the 20th day of pregnancy

Prenatal cholinergic drug exposure to pregnant females resulted in sex-linked alterations of the brain dopaminergic and serotoninergic systems. Whereas the brain dopaminergic system of genotypical males and famales embryos was more sensitive to influence of N-cholinotropic drug ganglerone.

Neurochemical data analysis of the neurotransmitter status of the rats embryos brain of a various genetical sex has shown that prenatal influence by cholinolytics of the central action - methylbenactyzine and ganglerone– in case of injection on 9-19 days of the gestation causes a disbalance in the content of neurotransmitters of DA, 5-HT and their metabolites in the embryos brain of experimental groups by 20 day of prenatal development in comparison with control.

4.1 Metabolism of dopamine

Males embryos have a weaker density of DA (fig. 3) after prenatal ganglerone exposure on 9-11 days of prenatal development (G10 group). Level of DOPAC (dihydroxy-phenyl acetic acid), DA metabolite, did not change (tab. 2) during the same period. In G10 group decrease of the DA content was accompanied by augmentation of its turnover. At ganglerone introduction on 12-14 days of gestation was noted a substantial growth of DA level (on 29,9 %, p <0,01) which was not accompanied by change of its turnover that testifies the augmentation of mediatory synthesis intensity.

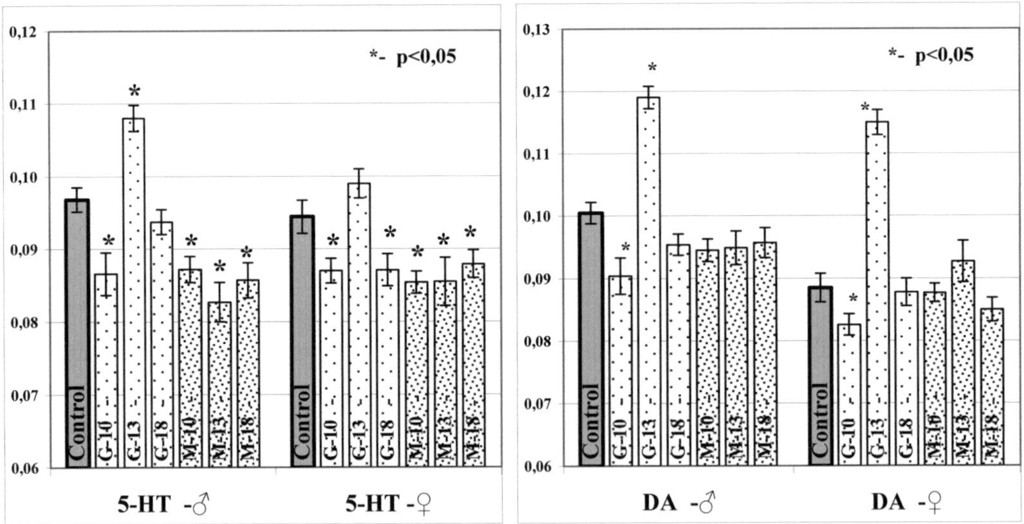

*-p < 0.05 compared with the control group. For further details see caption to Fig. 1.

Fig. 3. Content of dopamine and serotonine (ng/mg of wet tissue) in the Brains of 20-day rat embryos. Notations: - ♂, - ♀ - signs of genotypical males and famales embryos.

Females embryos in groups with prenatal ganglerone exposure on 9-11 days of prenatal development also had authentic decrease of DA concentration and its useful increase (on 18,4 %, p≤0,01) after drug introduction on 12-14 day of gestation. At the same time fameles had more sugnificant change of DOPAC content. It was also noticed that in contrast to males, females embryos change of DA level was accompanied by more appreciable decrease of DA turnover in all experimental groups. The most appreciable decrease of DA/DOPAC ratio was reveled during early period of gestation after ganglerone exposure and during more late pregnancy after methylbenactyzine exposure.

4.2 Metabolism of serotonine

Alteration of 5-HT level in the embryonal brain was more considerable in comparison with DA. Thus in all investigated periods of gestation in comparison with control group authentically significant reduction of 5-HT content in the embryos brain by exposure of methylbenactyzine and ganglerone was noted.

It was noted that males embryos 5-HT concentration in the brain was sugnificantly decreased in all periods of prenatal methylbenactyzine exposure. In the G10-G18 groups significant decrease of 5-HT concentration in the embryos brain is noted at drug introduction on 9-11 and 17-19 days of prenatal development. Dynamics of 5-HIAA (5-hydroxyindoleacetic acid) content (metabolite of 5-HT) was similar to the mediator content, thus noted significant decrease in M10 - M13 and G10 groups.

The comparative analysis of the received data shows that in the prenatal period the serotoninergic transmitter system is more sensitive to exposure of cholinolytics than dopaminergic system. 5-HT concentration and its turnover decrease during the second half of gestation with influence of the methylbenactyzine , and the ganglerone. Whereas the brain dopaminergic system of genotypical males and females embryos is more sensitive to influence N-cholinergic antagonist ganglerone.

Many researches show the sensitivity of neurotransmitter system of a developing brain to influence of various drugs and ecological toxicants, possessing cholinergic activity. For example, the neurochemical alterations caused by the prenatal exposition of nicotine, are well studied; it is noticed that prenatally introduced nicotine damages development of the central mechanisms noradrenergic, dopaminergic, serotoninergic and cholinergic system in the rats brain (Lichtensteiger et al., 1988; Ribary & Lichtensteiger, 1989; King et al., 1991; Lichtensteiger & Schlumpf, 1993; Muneoka et al., 1997). Moreover, there is data that various reactions to prenatal exposure of nicotine are bound to a genetical sex of embryos (Genedani et al., 1983; Levin et al., 1993; Shacka et al., 1997).

Thus, prenatal cholinergic drug exposure produced dramatic imbalance of the neurotransmitter contents and turnover in the rat fetus brain on the 20th day of pregnancy. The comparative analysis showed that the serotoninergic neurotransmitter system was more sensitive to influence of cholinolytics in prenatal period than dopaminergic system. Decreasing of 5-HT concentration and its turnover in all «critical periods» on the second half of pregnancy was marked under influence as methylbenactyzine, and ganglerone, the M- and N-cholinolytics respectively. Whereas the brain dopaminergic system of genotypical males and famales embryos was more sensitive to influence of N-cholinotropic drug ganglerone. Thus, prenatal influence of cholinotropic drugs on pregnant females resulted in sex-linked alterations of brain dopaminergic and serotoninergic systems at 20-day's old fetuses of rats. These alterations can be involved to ethiopathogenesis of behavioral dysfunctions of rats progenies in pubertal period and be connected with deviant behavior.

groups	n	DOPAC -♂	5-HIAA -♂	DOPAC -♀	5-HIAA -♀
Control	**63**	0,0121+0,0008	0,1262+0,0030	0,0150+0,0011	0,1292+0,0031
G10	**33**	0,0132+0,0030	0,1139+0,0032	0,0054+0,0006*	0,1049+0,0034*
G13	**16**	0,0110+0,0013	0,1390+0,0042	0,0090+0,0009*	0,1280+0,0045
G18	**36**	0,0054+0,0004*	0,1278+0,0026	0,0102+0,0006*	0,1112+0,0019
M10	**41**	0,0085+0,0008*	0,1156+0,0028	0,0115+0,0008*	0,1116+0,0030
M13	**47**	0,0119+0,0004	0,1000+0,0025*	0,0097+0,0005*	0,1034+0,0030*
M18	**32**	0,0090+0,0009*	0,1061+0,0032	0,0051+0,0003*	0,1074+0,0025*

*-p < 0.05 compared with control group.

Table 2. Content of DOPAC and 5-HIAA in the brains of 20-day rat embryos. (M ± m)
Notations: - ♂, - ♀ - simbols of the genetical sex of offspring, accordingly males and females.

5. The long-term neurochemical effects of prenatal exposure to selective M- and N-cholinolytics

Prenatal exposure of some neurotropic agents results not only in disturbances of a proliferation and a differentiation of embryos brain neurones, but also causes the remote disorders of development of synaptic function of brain neurones, disturbance of ontogenetic development of the brain basic neurotransmitter systems in the postnatal period (Robinson, 2000; Icenogle, 2004). Studying of development of the central monoaminergic systems of the brain structures participating in regulation neuroendocrinal and behavioral functions of organism of the rats offspring aged 2 months, therefore is obviously important.

The investigations showed that the prenatal exposure of M- and N-cholinolytics to pregnant females produces long-term neurochemical changes in development of brain neuromediatory systems. In the investigated of brain structures, both at males, and at females of rats progenies, exposure to prenatal cholinolytics, significant decrease of DA, 5-HT, NA concentrations and change of level of their metabolites is marked.

The analysis of the received data has shown that prenatal introduction of cholinolytics with selective M- and N-cholinergic activity (methylbenactyzine and ganglerone) to pregnant females leads to the remote changes of brain monoaminergic system activity (DA, NA and 5-HT) of 2-month-old rats offspring.

5.1 Hippocampus

Rats offrspins that were subjected to prenatal exposure of a ganglerone had a decreased in 1,5 - 2,5 times (p≤0,001) DA level in the hippocampus. The greatest falling of DA level noted

in group with ganglerone exposure on 9-11 days of a gestation (fig. 4). Though in groups with prenatal exposure of a methylbenactyzine DA content in a hippocampus has not changed. In group M10 among offsprings with a prenatal exposition of a methylbenactyzine was noted a tendency to augmentation.
Dynamics of DOPAC in the studied groups in comparison to control groups was opposite to DA content - substantial growth of DOPAC concentration in groups G10 and G13 (accordingly on 21,7 % and 26,3 %, p≤0,001) was noted. The neurochemical status in hippocampus of the males prenatally exposured to cholinolytics was characterized by serious decrease of DA concentration and change of its metabolite level in comparison with control offsprings.

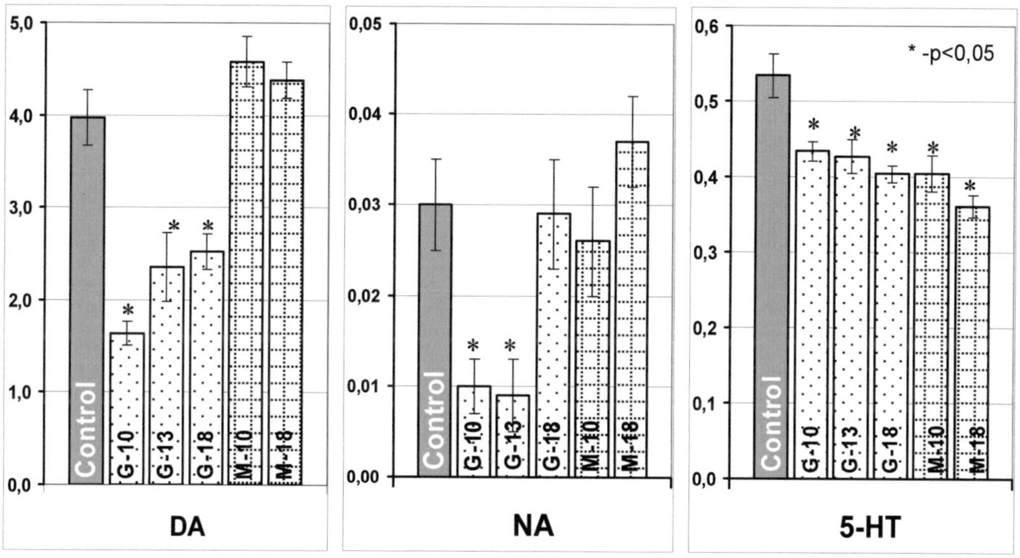

Fig. 4. Contents of dopamine (DA), noradrenaline (NA), and serotonine (5-HT) (ng/mg of wet tissue) in the hippocampus in two-month-old rat offspring exposed to methylbenactyzine or ganglerone at different periods of prenatal development. *p < 0.05 compared with the control group. For further details see caption to Fig. 1.

5.1.1 NA metabolism

The obtained data showed decrease of the NA content and increase of its metabolite MHPG (3-methoxy-4-hydroxyphenylethylene glycol) concentration that led to NA synaptic activity decrease. In case of rats males decrease of NA concentration in hippocampus was noted only in two groups subjected to prenatal exposure of a ganglerone in early periods of gestation - G10 and G13 (accordingly 66,6 % and 70,0 %, p≤0,001). Thus the content of a noradrenaline metabolite of MHPG has been enlarged in all investigated groups in 1,5 - 2,0 times.

5.1.2 5-HT metabolism

Unlike other neurotransmitters 5-HT level in the hippocampus has been reduced in all groups of both gender in comparison with control offsprings group. Males offsprings had significant reduction of 5-HT content in the range from 19,7 % (p≤0,01) - in G10 and to 32,6 % (p≤0,001) in M18 group. The serotonin metabolite level 5-HIAA in the hippocampus also has been reduced in groups with prenatal exposure of methylbenactyzine and ganglerone. Ratio indexes 5-HIAA/5-HT have been increased only in those groups in which decrease of mediator level became perceptible.

groups	HIPPOCAMPUS		HYPOTHALAMUS	
	DA	**5-HT**	**DA**	**5-HT**
Control	0,244±0,018	0,976±0,068	0,637±0,037	0,608±0,035
G-10	0,228±0,026	1,120±0,061	0,470±0,023*	0,578±0,041
G-13	0,194±0,022	1,192±0,078*	0,461±0,030*	0,636±0,028
G-18	0,340±0,020*	1,134±0,062*	0,540±0,026	0,587±0,032
M-10	0,344±0,022*	1,240±0,059*	0,378±0,033*	0,538±0,039
M-18	0,402±0,031*	1,188±0,069*	0,490±0,041*	0,550±0,039

Table 3. Turnover of DA and 5-HT neurotransmitters in hippocampus and hypothalamus at 2-month-old rat offspring exposed to methylbenactyzine or ganglerone at different periods of prenatal development. (M ± m) *-p < 0.05 compared with the control group

Research of neurotransmitters turnover in the hippocampus has shown that rats offspring subjected to exposure of cholinolytics have an enchancement of the turnover of the basic mediators, leading to decrease of concentration of these neurotransmitters in the hippocampus. Noted increase of DA turnover in the hippocampus of rats offspring prenatally subjected to exposure by methylbenactyzine (tab. 3) and significant increase of 5-HT turnover in the hippocampus of the offsprings, subjected to prenatal exposure both methylbenactyzine and ganglerone.

5.2 Hypothalamus

5.2.1 DA metabolism

The neurochemical status of DA in the hypothalamus of 2-month-old rats offsprings subjected to prenatal exposure of cholinolytics, was characterised by significant decrease of dopaminergic activity in relation to control (fig. 5). In comparison with the methylbenactyzine, prenatal exposure of the ganglerone, caused more appreciable remote changes of DA level in the hypothalamus of these offsprings.

Concentration of the DA has been reduced in all groups - G10 - G18 (31,7 % - 36,9 %, p≤0,001) with maximally low value in G13 group. Among offsprings with prenatal exposure to methylbenactyzine significant decrease of DA noted only in M18 group (17,6 %, p≤0,05). Dynamics of DOPAC change in relation to control group was similar to dynamics of DA significant 1,5 - 2 times decrease of DOPAC concentration in all groups was noted.

5.2.2 NA metabolism

The neurochemical status of NA in the hypothalamus was characterised by rising of processes of degradation of a mediator without enchancement of synthesis processes. In all studied groups both males and females had a decreased NA level and high MHPG content in the hypothalamus in comparison with control offsprings' grou. In comparison with methylbenactyzine, NA concentration in groups with prenatal exposure to ganglerone, has been reduced more considerably (in a greater degree in G10 group - decrease of the NA of 26,2 %, p≤0,001). The content of MHPG metabolite, on the contrary, has been raised in all groups in 1,5 - 2,5 times.

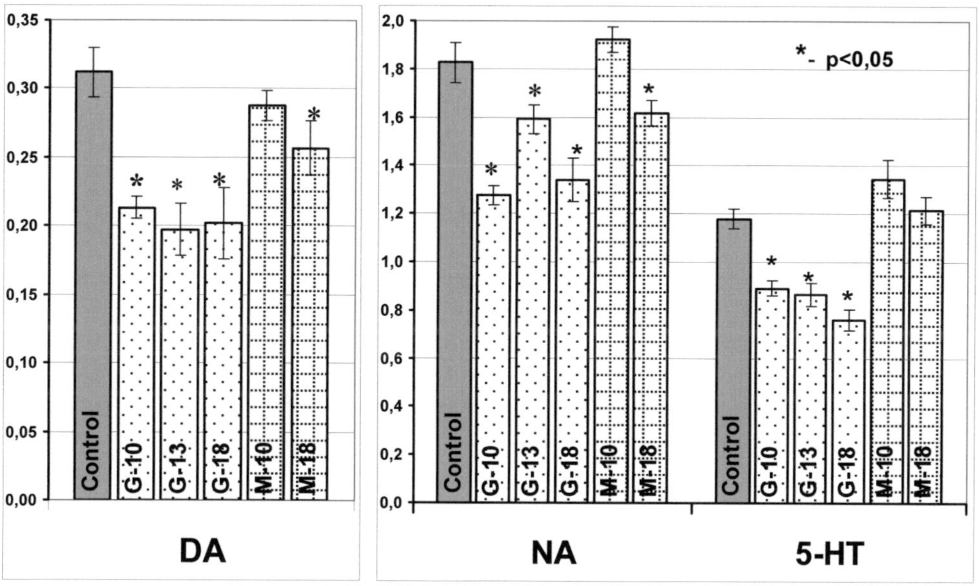

Fig. 5. Contents of dopamine (DA), noradrenaline (NA), and serotonin (5-HT) (ng/mg of wet tissue) in the hypothalamus in two-month-old rat offspring exposed to methylbenactyzine or ganglerone at different periods of prenatal development. *p < 0.05 compared with the control group. For further details see caption to Fig. 1.

5.2.3 5-HT metabolism

Dynamics of 5-HT change in the hypothalamus was similar to other mediators – rats offsprings from G10 - G18 groups, where mediator level has been reduced in significant limens (accordingly, 24,3 % - 35,4 %, p≤0,001), had more radical changes in 5-HT content in G10 - G18 groups. In methylbenactyzine groups 5-HT concentration in the hypothalamus strengthened (in M10 group on 14,2 %, p≤0,05). 5-HIAA metabolite content in the hypothalamus of all the studied groups was similar to dynamics of the mediator.

The greatest changes of the neurotransmitters turnover in the hypothalamus have been detected concerning a DA both of rats males and females (tab. 1). DA turnover has considerably reduced in the males hypothalamus in all experimental groups in comparison with control group. The ratio index 5-HIAA/5-HT was more stable, except for G10 group of females which index was reduced. In the same group increase of 5-HT level at the stable content 5-HIAA was noticed that shows enchancement of serotoninergic synaptic activity in the hypothalamus. NA turnover in the hypothalamus of experimental groups was comparable with the data of control group though the mediator content and its metabolite has been reduced in all groups.

Sexual dimorphism in effects of prenatal exposure of M- and N-cholinolytics on dopaminergic system (fig.6) has been detected. In case of males offspring that were exposed to prenatal exposure of a ganglerone N-cholinolitics the decrease of DA concentration in the brain structures was noted; in case of rats females - the same reduction after prenatal exposure to M-cholinolytic methylbenactyzine.

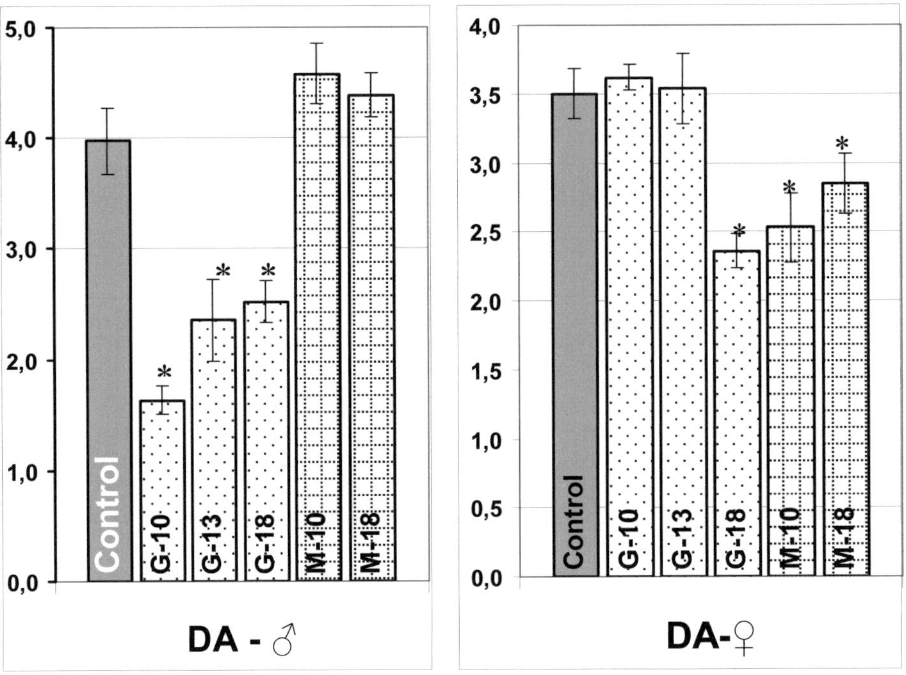

Fig. 6. Sexual dimorphism according to dophamine concentration (ng/mg of wet tissue) in the hippocampus in two-month-old rat offspring exposed to methylbenactyzine or ganglerone at different periods of prenatal development. $*p<0.05$ compared with the control group. Notations: - ♂, - ♀ - simbols of the genetical sex of offspring, accordingly males and females.

5.3 Amygdala

For realization of adaptive and sexual behavior dopaminergic system of amygdala is also important. The amygdala initiates the organization of adequate behavior to the situation and by means of influence on the hypothalamus and vegetative excitatory system frames conforming hormonal and neurovegetative assurance to this behavior (Simonov, 1987). According to many researchers an amygdaloid complex is responsible for integration of emotional expressions, characteristic for sexual motivation (Newman, 1999; Dominguez, 2001).

Dynamics of neurotransmitters level in the amygdala was similar to the neurochemical status in the hippocampus that once again confirms their morphophysiologycal generality within limbic system. Long-term effects of prenatal exposures of cholinolytics within amygdala nuclei have been brightly expressed. Study's results show significant decrease of DA, 5-HT and NA mediators content in the amygdala of the males prenatally subjected to exposure of gangleron, larger degree on 10-13 days of gestation (fig. 7). Prenatal exposure of M-cholinolytic methylbenactyzine had no strongly pronounced consequences on development of neurotransmitter systems in the amygdala

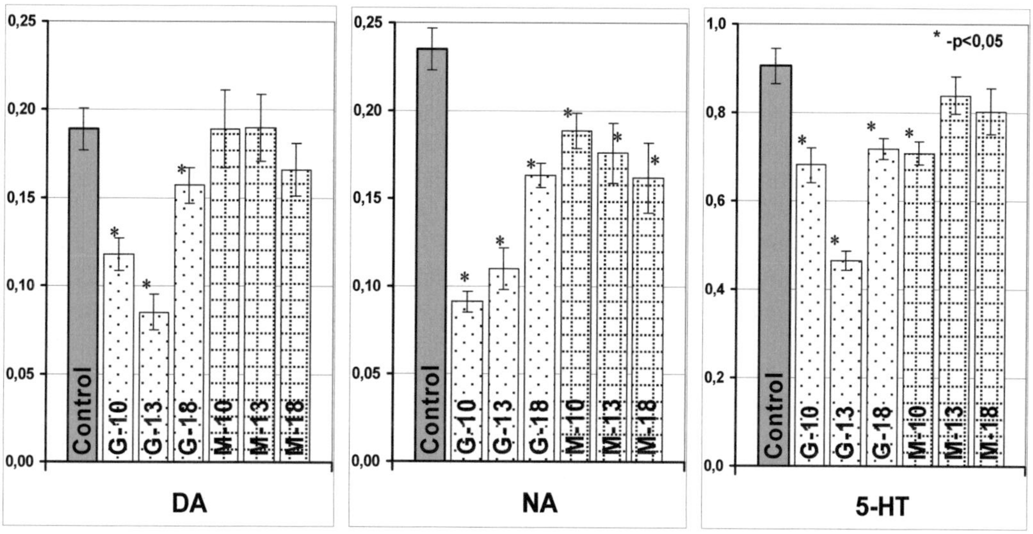

Fig. 7. Contents of dopamine (DA), noradrenaline (NA), and serotonin (5-HT) (ng/mg of wet tissue) in the amygdala in two-month-old rat offspring exposed to methylbenactyzine or ganglerone at different periods of prenatal development. *p < 0.05 compared with the control group. For further details see caption to Fig. 1.

Changes of the neurotrasmitter status in the amygdala can affect functioning of other brain structures participating in regulation of sexual function, by means of neuronal connection of this structure with hippocampus and hypothalamus. It is shown that destruction of hypothalamo-amigdaloid connection, damage or irritation of the amygdala lead to neurohumoral alterations and sexual behavior abnormalities (Akmaev, 1993; Swanson, 1998; Dominguez, 2001). It is not excluded that optimization of integrative connections within limbic system and hypothalamus is extremely important concerning the effects of cholinergic system on sexual function.

Results of these researches show that pregnant females in "critical periods" of the embryo prenatal development exposure to M- and N-cholinoblockers can cause long-term changes in neurotransmitter systems activity in investigated structures of the rats brain in their postnatal life.

Exposure of M- and N-cholinolytics in the prenatal period leads to significant decrease of dopaminergic activity in the hippocampus and hypothalamus of rats offspring in comparison with control group. Results of various researches prove that defects of DA synaptic activity in the hippocampus at offspring can accompany to hippocampus-associated behavioral deficiencies at puberal individuals (Yanai, 1984; Smith, et al. 1986; Steingart et al., 2000).

The prenatal nicotine exposure which is exogenous ligand of N-cholinergic receptor leads to nonperishable change of activity of the basic neurotransmitter systems in brain structures in a postnatal period. The decrease of DA concentration in the brain structures at males has been detected at offspring which were subjected to prenatal exposure of N-cholinolytic ganglerone, and at females - to mainly prenatal exposure of M-cholinolytic methylbenactyzine (Genedani et al., 1983; Ribary, 1985; Lichtensteiger et al., 1988; Lichtensteiger & Schlumpf, 1993; Muneoka et al., 1997).

In spite of various mechanisms of M- and N-cholinolytics action in the organism, the long-term effects of these drugs on the basic transmitter systems development in offspring are basically the same, namely inhibiting a metabolism of these neurotransmitters. Prenatal exposure of selective M- and N-cholinolytics, like other chemical drugs and ecological toxicants with cholinergic properties, causes the long-term changes in programming of neurotransmitter functions in 2-month's offspring which, in turn, can participate in the development of neuro-behavioral anomalies, appetent and affective disturbances at puberal individuals (Lauder, 1985; Turlejski, 1996; Levitt et al., 1997; Dreyfus, 1998; Azmitia, 2001).

Thus, the prenatal exposure of M- and N-cholinolytics to pregnant females produces long-term neurochemical changes in the development of brain neuromediatory systems. In the studied brain structures, both males and females, exposure to prenatal cholinolytics, significant decrease of DA, 5-HT, NA concentrations and change of level of their metabolites were marked. Prenatal exposure to ganglerone N-cholinolytics to pregnant females on 9-19 gestational days exerts most appreciable long-term effect on neurotransmitter development, which leads to reduction of dopaminergic, noradrenergic and serotonergic activity in the hippocampus and hypothalamus of 2-month-old rats progenies in comparison with control group. Is was noted that prenatal exposure of cholinolytics on DA concentration in the brain structures at 2-month-old rats progenies causes sexual dimorphism. These results indicate that exposure to M- and N-cholinolytics during the critical periods of prenatal development (9-11 and 12-14 gestational days) results in long-term changes in development of neuromediatory systems in the brain structure, which participate in regulation of behavioral and neuroendocrinal functions of rats offsprings.

6. Endocrinological consequences of prenatal exposure to N-cholinolytics in the rats offspring's

The involvement of N-cholinergic mechanisms in behavioral impairments in male offspring is associated with the properties of N-cholinoreceptors, which are involved in the regulation of the catecholaminergic system of the CNS. N-cholinergic neurons are connected to different types of neurons in the brain, and activation of N-cholinoreceptors by endogenous (acetylcholine) or exogenous (nicotine) ligands modulates the release of the transmitters DA, NA, and 5-HT, depending on the type of cell (Retana, 1993; McGehee et al., 1995). Nicotinic receptors are abundant in the subcortical areas of the brain during early fetal development (Lisk & Greemvald, 1983), so embryonic exposure to nicotine damages noradrenergic and dopaminergic synaptic transmission in the brain (Navarro et al., 1988; Seidler et al., 1992).

It follows from this that the mechanism of prenatal exposure to the N-cholinolytic ganglerone on sexual function in offspring may be mediated by modulation of brain transmitter systems, including DA, NA, and 5-HT systems, which indirectly regulate the processes of motivation and components of coitus (Bitran & Hull, 1987; Gladkova, 2000; Mas et al., 1987; Pfaus & Phillips, 1991). This thesis is supported by results from neurochemical studies, which have demonstrated that administration of an N-cholinolytic to pregnant females at different periods of gestation leads to long-term changes in the development of brain neurotransmitter systems in 20-day embryos and two-month offspring of rats.

The most significant changes in the concentrations of DA, 5-HT, and NA and their metabolites in brain structures were seen after administration of ganglerone at 9–11 and 12–14 days of gestation, which was apparent as reductions in the synaptic activities of these brain neurotransmitter systems, particularly dopaminergic activity in the hippocampus and hypothalamus in two-month-old offspring of rats as compared with controls. Although 20-day embryos showed an increase in DA levels in response to administration of ganglerone at 12–14 days of gestation, this requires further investigation. It can be suggested that like nicotine, ganglerone, blocking N-cholinergic receptors, induced impairments to the formation and establishment of network systems in the developing embryonic brain, which promoted stable decreases in the synaptic activity of the transmitter systems of interest in the hippocampus and hypothalamus of twomonth-old offspring rats as compared with controls. This imbalance in neurotransmitter activity in brain limbic structures in two-month-old offspring is a long-term neurochemical effect of prenatal treatment with ganglerone, which in turn may facilitate sexual dysfunction in fertile males.

The neurotransmitter DA plays an important role in activating the sexual behavior in male rats; DA depletion in brain structures involved in regulating the behavioral states of body facilitates reductions in sexual activity (Gladkova, 2000; Mas et al., 1987; Pfaus & Phillips, 1991). Lesioning of different dopaminergic projections induces different behavioral syndromes depending on which part of the CNS is lesioned (Carey & Schwarting, 1986; Simon et al., 1986); in particular, damage to the dopaminergic projections of limbic structures leads to impairments in male sexual function (Hull et al., 1984).

The noradrenergic and serotoninergic systems of the brain are also involved in regulating hormone-dependent behavioral states, including sexual behavior (Naumenko et al., 1983; Lenahan et al., 1986; Smeets & Reiner, 1994). Affecting the secretion of gonadoliberin in the hypothalamic nuclei, NA and 5-HT act on $\alpha 2,\beta 2$-adrenoreceptors and 5-HT1,2 serotonin receptors to take part in the central regulation of the endocrine system of the male body and, thus, in controlling male sexual function.

Thus, prenatal modulation of N-cholinergic brain mechanisms with ganglerone can alter the activities of DA, NA, and 5-HT systems, which are directly involved in regulating motivation and components of coitus in adult offspring. We believe that this mechanism is the main cause of long-term behavioral impairments in pubescent offspring subjected to prenatal exposure to cholinolytics. The prenatal effects of cholinolytics on sexual function in offspring represent a paradox, which is that in relation to the cholinergic system, sexual activity in adult males is regulated mainly by M-cholinolytic mechanisms, while during the prenatal period, these are more dependent on the activity of N-cholinergic system.

Another mechanism mediating the long-term actions of cholinolytics on sexual function in offspring consists of the involvement of endocrine factors. Considering the role of the central and peripheral compartments of the nervous system in controlling the hypothamalo-hypophyseal-gonadal system in males, it can be suggested that prenatal administration of cholinolytics to pregnant females might also have long-term consequences in relation to the endocrine system of offspring.

The results obtained from endocrine studies supported the occurrence of endocrine impairments in pubescent offspring (Fig. 8). A significant reduction in testosterone levels was seen in offspring subjected to prenatal exposure to ganglerone at different periods of gestation, with lowest values seen in the offspring of group G13 (2.4-fold decrease). There was also a significant decrease in the testosterone level in offspring subjected to prenatal exposure to methylbenactyzine in group M18. The LH and FSH levels in the blood of all groups were increased.

The hormonal-motivational component of sexual behavior of male rats is known to controlled at the central level by testosterone, which is metabolized to estradiol, while ejaculation is controlled at the peripheral level by the non-aromatized dihydrotestosterone and only partially by testosterone (Lisk, 1983). Low testosterone levels in G10–G13 offspring could therefore facilitate alterations in both the central motivational and the peripheral ejaculatory components of sexual behavior. The reduced testosterone level in G10–G18 offspring correlated with low sexual activity and, conversely, numbers of the sexually more active males of groups M10–M18 had higher testosterone levels.

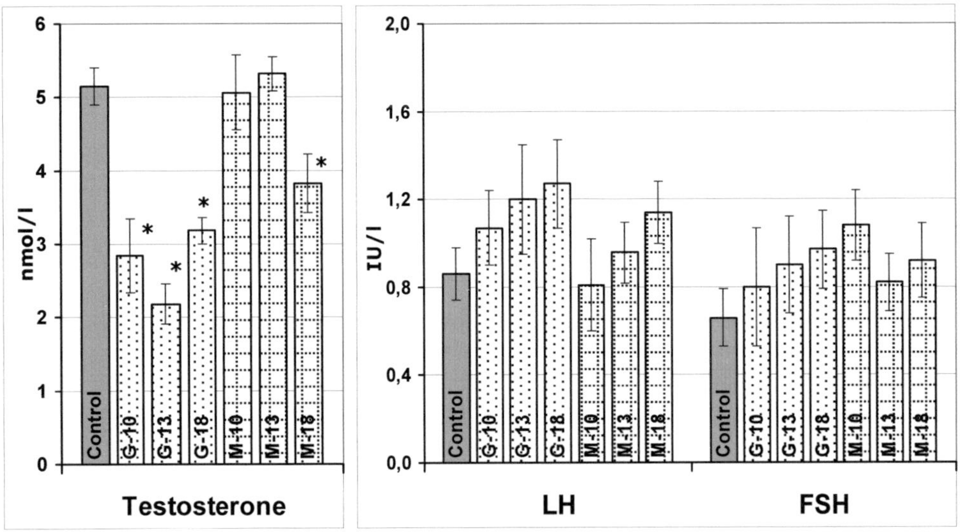

Fig. 8. Serum Testosterone, LH and FSH levels in two-month-old rat offspring exposed to ganglerone or methylbenactyzine at different periods of prenatal development. *p < 0.05 compared with control group. For further details see caption to Fig. 1.

Thus, along with neuronal factors, changes in the hormonal background probably represent a further cause of impairments to sexual functions in offspring subjected to prenatal exposure to central cholinolytics. Reproductive impairments induced by damage to the neuroendocrine and neurotransmitter systems during the fetal period of ontogenesis due to prenatal exposure to cholinolytics may in later life become the cause of impairments to the ability of males to mate and produce offspring.

7. Correction of sexual dysfunction of the males subjected to influence of selective cholinolytics in the early prenatal period

The studies showed that rat males characterized by low sexual activity, were very sensitive to effects of agonists of the cholinergic and dopaminergic systems. The correction of sexual activity was observed only during the period of action of these drugs and did not appear in delayed period after treatment.

Experimental researches have shown that the rats males subjected to prenatal exposure of a ganglerone and characterized by low sexual activity, have appeared sensitive to effects of cholinergic and dopaminergic (tab. 4).

G13 group		Mounts (n)	latency of mount (sec)	Intromissions (n)	latency of intromission (sec)	Ejaculation (n)	latency of ejaculation (sec)	Interejaculatory interval (sec)
Control		17,1 ±3,1	26,0 ±9,0	11,4 ±2,1	53,9 ±16,0	0,90 ±0,17	278,8 ±53,0	403,5 ±29,1
Arecoline	1 hour	29,6 ±1,3*	13,3 ±2,0*	17,1 ±2,9*	29,5 ±3,2*	1,83 ±0,22*	184,4 ±36,4*	313,4 ±41,2*
	7 days	14,1 ±2,1	21,9 ± 3,8	10,1 ±2,9	42,3 ±7,8	1,04 ±0,18	267,0 ±41,5	394,1 ±54,3
Galantamine + Ganglerone	1 hour	24,6 ±2,8*	12,4 ±2,5*	18,8 ±3,1*	28,7 ±4,7*	1,55 ±0,19*	198,3 ±36,0*	329,1 ±39,5*
	7 days	16,6 ±2,1	30,5 ± 4,1	12,0 ± 2,4	55,8 ±7,2	1,10 ±0,17	288,2 ±41,5	386,0 ±50,6
Apomorphinum	1 hour	31,6 ±4,4*	8,30 ±2,3*	21,2 ±3,8*	23,3 ±5,9*	1,97 ±0,30*	166,2 ±32,1*	320,5 ±52,6*
	7 days	19,9 ±3,0	24,2 ± 3,6	12,2 ±1,2	45,4 ±6,7	1,09 ±0,18	237,3 ±38,2	425,0 ±57,9

*-$p < 0.05$ compared with control group.
Note: The sexual activity is recorded in 1 hour after an injection and for 7 days of an afteraction of drugs.

Table 4. Parameters of sexual behavior in the mature male rats subjected to prenatal exposure to ganglerone on 12-14 day of gestation (G13 group) before and after application of the agents. (M±m).

Cholinomimetic drug arecoline (2 mg/kg), galantamine with a ganglerone (accordingly, 1mg/kg and 5 mg/kg) and agonist of D_1,D_2-dopaminergic receptors apomorphinum (1 mg/kg) considerably enhanced sexual function. Components of sexual function - mounts, intromissions and ejaculations after pharmacological correction were high enough though did not reach in certain cases indexes of sexual behavior of control offspring. On the contrary, time components of a sexual behavior specified about sufficient high degree of sexual activation, including motivation enchancement.
In spite of significant enchancement of the sexual function, the obtained data have shown that correction of sexual activity descended only during the period of drugs action - within 1 days. For 7 day after introduction of stimulating drugs quantitative and qualitative characteristics of rats male sexual behavior were reverted on initial level.

Prenatal exposure of cholinolytics also promoted appearance of high sensitivity of sexual function of offspring to effects of antagonists cholinergic and dopaminergic systems. The methylbenactyzine (3 mg/kg) and haloperidolum (0,5 mg/kg) in the doses depressing sexual activity of intact rats only to 50 %, completely quenched implication of sexual function at offspring G10, G13 and M10 groups.
Thus, the research results show that sexual dysfunction of the offspring subjected to prenatal exposure of M- and N-cholinolytics is a persistent sexual function abnormality that demands long courses of pathogenetic treatment.

8. Conclusions

- Results of the investigations show that prenatal exposure by ganglerone and methylbenactyzine leads to the delayed behavioral disturbances, significant and stable failure of sexual function of puberal males offspring. Ganglerone administration to pregnant females on 10-13 days of gestation has led to violent decrease of sexual function at puberal males, low level of ejaculatory components of sexual behavior with long enough stage of ejaculation latency. Significant damage of the motivational component, high latence of mount and intromissions of offspring in G10 and G13 groups was detected. Change of sexual activity of offspring with methylbenactyzine exposure have been less expressed, and after acquisition of sexual experience, these changes in comparison with control were levelled.
- The certain paradox in effect of cholinergic drugs on sexual function of males was noted: sexual activity of males is regulated by M-cholinergic system and prenatally depends on activity of N-cholinergic system. Neurotransmitter dysfunction of fertile 2-month-old males that were prenatally administered with cholinolytics predetermines predetermines behavioural disturbances, in particular sexual dysfunction of puberal offspring.
- Analysis of the received neurochemical data of the brain neurotransmitter status of 20-day-old embryos of a various genetical sex have shown that prenatal administration of cholinergic drugs of the central action type (methylbenactyzine and ganglerone) in different periods of gestation, causes a disbalance of the content of DA and 5-HT neurotransmitters and their metabolites in the embryos brain on 20 day of prenatal development in comparison with control group.
- Results of the experiments show that modulation of activity by M-cholinergic and N-cholinergic systems of a developing foetus brain can lead to significant changes in activity of the basic transmitter systems of an embryonal brain. Accordingly, mechanisms of prenatal exposure of various chemical factors with cholinergic properties can be mediated both M-cholinergic and N-cholinergic system.
- In the prenatal period the serotoninergic transmitter system is more sensitive to exposure of cholinolytics than dopaminergic system. The serotoninergic transmitter system is more sensitive to exposure of methylbenactyzine and ganglerone. The brain dopaminergic system of genotypical males and females embryos is more sensitive to N-cholinolytic ganglerone exposure.
- Exposure of pregnant females in "critical periods" of prenatal embryo development to M- and N-cholinoblockers caused long-term changes in activity of neurotransmitter systems in brain structures of 2-month-old rats offspring. Significant decrease of DA, 5-HT, NA concentration and change of level of their metabolites in the brain structures

participating in regulation of behavioral and neuroendocrinal functions of organism was detected.

- The most significant effect of ganglerone administration on neurotransmitter development was noted on 10-13 days of gestation when it led to decrease of synaptic activity of transmitter systems and growth of dopaminergic activity in the hippocampus and hypothalamus of 2-month-old rats offspring in comparison with control group.
- Change of hormonal background and significant decrease of the testosterone level in comparison with control offsprings' group is one of the causes of the reduced sexual function at the offspring subjected to prenatal ganglerone exposure. Low level of testosterone correlated with low sexual activity and high quantity of sexually inactive males in the same groups.
- Pharmacological correction of the reduced sexual activity descends only during a period of action of stimulating drugs. For 7 days after administration of stimulating drugs quantitative and qualitative characteristics of sexuality of rats males were reverted on basic level.

Thus, administration of cholinergic drugs to rats in the prenatal period produces prolonged influence on the neurotransmitters level, sexual hormones and sexual activity in adulthood. The reproductive problems caused by injuries of neuroendocrine system during the fetal period can compromise the later success of mating as well as the capacity to generate descendants.

9. References

Agmo A. (1997) Male rat sexual behavior. *Brain Research Protocols.* Vol.1, pp. 203-209.

Akmaev I.G., Kalimulina A.B. (1993) Amygdaloid complex of brain: Functional morphology and neuroendocrinology. (in Russian). M

Azmitia E.C. (2001) Modern views on an ancient chemical: serotonin effects on cell proliferation, maturation, and apoptosis. *Brain Res Bull.* Vol.56, pp. 413–424.

Beer A., Slotkin T.A., Seidler F.J., Aldridge J.E., Yanai J. (2005) Nicotine Therapy in Adulthood Reverses the Synaptic and Behavioral Deficits Elicited by Prenatal Exposure to Phenobarbital. *Neuropsychopharmacology.* Vol.30, pp. 156–165.

Bitran D., Hull E. (1987) Pharmacological analysis of male rat sexual behavior. *Neurosci. Biobehav. Rev.* Vol.11, pp. 365–389.

Buzsaki, G. (1989). Two-stage model of memory trace formation: a role for "noisy" brain states. *Neuroscience;* Vol.31, pp. 551–570.

Carey R.J., Schwarting R. (1986) Spontaneous and drug induced locomotor activity after partial dopamine denervation of the ventral striatum. *Neuropsychobiol.* Vol.16, pp. 121-125.

Dani J.A., Heinemann S. (1996) Molecular and cellular aspects of nicotine abuse. *Neuron.* Vol.16, pp. 905–908..

Dominguez JM, Hull EM. (2001) Stimulation of the medial amygdala enhances medial preoptic dopamine release: implications for male rat sexual behavior. *Brain Res.* Vol.917, No.2, pp. 225-229.

Dorner G. (1989) Hormone-dependent brain development and neuroendocrine prophylaxis. *Exp. Clin. Endocrinol.* Vol.94, No.1/2, pp. 4-22.

Everitt B.J., Robbins T.W. (1997) Central cholinergic systems and cognition. *Ann. Rev. Psychol.* Vol.48, pp. 649–684.

Fergusson D.M., Woodward L.J., Horwood L.J. (1998) Maternal smoking during pregnancy and psychiatric adjustment in late adolescence. *Archiv. of General Psychiatry.* Vol.55, pp. 721-727.

Gladkova A.I. (1994) "Sexual differences in involutional changes in sexual behavior in rats," (in Russian) Probl. *Stareniya i Dolgoletiya.* Vol.4, pp. 322–333.

Gladkova A.I. (2000) Neuropharmacological Modification of Male Sexual Behavior in Rats. *Neurophysiology.* Vol.32, No.4, pp. 322-326.

Hull E.M., Bitran D., Pehek E., Holmes G., Warner R., Band L., Clemens L. (1988a) Brain localization of cholinergic influence on male sexual behavior in rats: agonists. *Pharmacol. Biochem. Behav.* Vol.31, pp. 169–174..

Hull E.M., Nishita J.K., Bitran D., Dalterio S. (1984) Perinatal dopamine-related drugs demasculinize rats. *Science.* Vol.224, No.4652, pp. 1011-1013.

Hull E.M., Pehek E., Bitran D., Holmes G., Warner R., Band L., Bazzet T., Clemens L. (1988b) Brain localization of cholinergic influence of male sexual behavior: antagonists. *Pharmacol. Biochem. Behav.* Vol.31, pp. 175–178.

Le Douarin NM. (1981) Plasticity in the development of the peripheral nervous system. *Ciba Symp;* Vol.83, pp. 19- 46.

Lenahan S.E., Siebel H.R., Jonson J.H. (1986) Evidence for multiple serotoninergic influence on LH release in ovariectomized rats and for modulation of their relative effectiveness by estrogen. *Neuroendocrinology.* Vol.44, No.1, pp. 89-94.

Levin E.D., S.J. Briggs, N.C. Christopher, J.E. Rose, (1993). Prenatal nicotine exposure and cognitive performance in rats, *Neurotoxicol. Teratol.* Vol.15, pp. 251-260.

Levin E.D., Simon B.B. (1998) Nicotinic acetylcholine involvement in cognitive function in animals. *Psychopharmacology.* Vol.138, pp. 217–230.

Levin E.D., Slotkin T.A. (1998) *Developmental neurotoxicity of nicotine.* Academic Press: San Diego.

Lichtensteiger W., Ribary U., Schlumpf M., Odermatt B., Widmer H.R. (1988) Prenatal adverse effects of nicotine on the developing brain. *Prog. Brain Res.* Vol.73, pp. 137–157.

Lisk R.D., Greemvald D.P. (1983) Central plus peripheral stimulation by androgen is necessary for complete restoration of copulatory behavior in the male hamster. *Neuroendocrinology.* Vol.36, No.3, pp. 211-214.

Mas M., Rodrıguez C., Guerra M., Guerra M., Davidson J., Battaner E. (1987) Neurochemical correlates of male sexual behavior. *Physiol. Behav.* Vol.41, pp. 341–345.

McGehee D.S., Heath M.J., Gelber S. Gelber S., Devay R., Role L.W. (1995) Nicotine enhancement of fast excitatory synaptic transmission in CNS by presynaptic receptors. *Science.* Vol.269, pp. 1692-1696.

Milberger, S., Biederman, J., Faraone, S.V., Chen, L., and Jones, J. (1996). Is maternal smoking during pregnancy a risk factor for attention deficit hyperactivity disorder in children? *American Journal of Psychiatry,* Vol.153, pp. 1138-1142.

Naeye, R.L. and Peters, E.C. (1984). Mental development of children whose mothers smoked during pregnancy. *Obstetrics and Gynecology,* Vol.64, pp. 601 - 607.

Naumenko E.V., Osadchuk A.V., Serova L.I., Shishkina G. T. (1983) *Genetik-physiological mechanisms of regulation of Testicular Function* (in Russian), Nauka, Novosibirsk.

Navarro H.A., Seidler F.J., Whitmore W.L., Slotkin T.A. (1988) Prenatal exposure to nicotine via maternal infusions: effects on development of catecholamine systems. *J. Pharmacol. Exp. Ther.* Vol.244, pp. 940–944.

Newman SW. (1999) The medial extended amygdala in male reproductive behavior. A node in the mammalian social behavior network. *Ann N Y Acad Sci.* Vol.877, pp. 242-57.

Nicholls, K. Psychotropics. In: Rubin, P. (Ed.), (2000) *Prescribing in pregnancy.* London: BMJ Books.

Oliff HS, Gallardo KA. (1999) The effect of nicotine on developing brain catecholamine systems. *Front Biosci.* Vol.4, pp. 883-897.

Orlebeke J.F., Knol D.L., Verhulst F.C. (1997) Increase in child behavior problems resulting from maternal smoking during pregnancy. *Arch. Environ. Health.* Vol.52, pp. 317-321.

Pendleton RG, Rasheed A, Roychowdhury R, Hillman RA. (1998) New role for catecholamines: ontogenesis. *Trends Pharmacol Sci.* Vol.19, pp. 248– 51.

Peters D.A.V. (1986) Prenatal stress increases the behavioral response to serotonin agonists and alters open field behavior in the rat. *Pharmacol. Biochem. Behav.* Vol..25, pp. 873-877.

Pfaus J.G., Phillips A.G. (1991) Role of dopamine in anticipatory and consummatory aspects of sexual behavior in the male rat. *Behav. Neurosci.* Vol.105, pp. 727–743.

Qiao D, Seidler F.J, Abreu-Villaзa Y, Tate C.A, Cousins M.M, Slotkin T.A. (2004) Chlorpyrifos exposure during neurulation: cholinergic synaptic dysfunction and cellular alterations in brain regions at adolescence and adulthood. *Dev. Brain Res.* Vol.148. P.43–52.

Qiao D, Seidler FJ, Padilla S, Slotkin TA. (2002) Developmental neurotoxicity of chlorpyrifos: what is the vulnerable period? *Environ. Health Perspect.* Vol.110, pp. 1097–1103.

Retana S., Domınguez E., Velazquez-Moctezuma J. (1993) Muscarinic and nicotinic influences on masculine sexual behavior in rats. *Pharmacol. Biochem. Behav.* Vol.44, pp. 913–917.

Seidler F.J., Levin E.D., Lappi S.E., Slotkin T.A. (1992) Fetal nicotine exposure ablates the ability of postnatal nicotine challenge to release norepinephrine from rat brain regions. *Dev. Brain Res.* Vol.69, pp. 288–291.

Sherman K.A., Kuster J.E., Dean R.L., Bartus R.T., Friedman E. (1981) Presynaptic cholinergic mechanisms in brain of aged rats with cognitive impairment. *Neurobiol. Aging.* Vol.2, pp. 99–104.

Simon H., Taghzouti K., Le Moal M. (1986) Deficits in spatial-memory tasks following lesions of septal dopaminergic terminals in the rat. *Behav. Brain Res.* Vol.19, No.1, pp. 7-16.

Simonov PV (1987) *A motivational brain.* (in Russian) M: Nauka,

Slotkin T.A. (2002) Functional alterations in CNS catecholamine systems in adolescence and adulthood after neonatal chlorpyrifos exposure. *Dev. Brain Res.* Vol.133, pp. 163–173.

Slotkin T.A. (2004) Cholinergic systems in brain development and disruption by neurotoxicants: nicotine, environmental tobacco smoke, organophosphates. *Toxicol. Appl. Pharmacol.* Vol.198, pp. 132-151.

Slotkin T.A., Cousins M.L., Tate C.A., Seidler F.J. (2001) Persistent cholinergic presynaptic deficits after neonatal chlorpyrifos exposure. *Brain Res.* Vol.902, pp. 229-243.

Smeets W.J., Reiner A. (1994) *Catecholamines in the CNS of vertebrates: current concepts of evolution and functional significance.* University Press, Cambridge.

Smith D.B, Goldstein S.G, Roomet A. (1986) A comparison of the toxicity effects of the anticonvulsant eterobarb (antilon, DMMP) and phenobarbital in normal human volunteers. *Epilepsia.* Vol.27, pp. 149–155.

Steingart R.A, Abu-Roumi M, Newman ME, Silverman WF, Slotkin TA, Yanai J. (2000) Neurobehavioral damage to cholinergic systems caused by prenatal exposure to heroin or phenobarbital: cellular mechanisms and the reversal of deficits by neural grafts. *Brain Res Dev Brain Res.* Vol.122, pp. 125–133.

Swanson L.W. (2000) Cerebral hemisphere regulation of motivated behavior. *Brain Res.* Vol.886, pp. 113–124.

Wallace S.J. (1984) *Studies on the Effect of Anticonvulsant Drugs on the Developing Human Brain.* Elsevier Science Publishers BV: Amsterdam. pp. 133–151.

Williams, G.M., O'Callaghan, M., Najman, J.M., Bor, W., Andersen, M.J., Richards, D. and Chunley, U. (1998). Maternal cigarette smoking and child psychiatric morbidity: a longitudinal study. *Pediatrics,* Vol.102, pp. e11.

Yanai J, Abu-Roumi M, Silverman W.F, Steingart R.A. (1996) Neural grafting as a tool for the study and reversal of neurobehavioral birth defects. *Pharmacol Biochem Behav.* Vol. 55, pp. 673–681.

Yanai J. (1984) An animal model for the effects of barbiturate on the development of the central nervous system. *Neurobehav. Terarol.* Vol.20, pp. 111–132.

Zoli M., Picciotto M.R., Ferrari R., Cocchi D., Changeux J.P. (1999) Increased neurodegeneration during ageing in mice lacking high-affinity nicotine receptors. *EMBO J.* Vol.18, pp. 1235–1244.

7

The Effects of Sildenafil Citrate on the Liver and Kidneys of Adult Wistar Rats (*Rattus norvegicus*) – A Histological Study

Andrew Osayame Eweka[1] and Abieyuwa Eweka[2]
[1]*Department of Anatomy, School of Basic Medical Sciences, College of Medical Sciences, University of Benin, Benin City, Edo State,*
[2]*School of Nursing, University of Benin Teaching Hospital, Benin City Edo State, Nigeria*

1. Introduction

Sildenafil citrate is widely used as an effective and safe oral treatment for erectile dysfunction of various etiologies (Goldstein et al., 1998; Cheitlin et al., 1999; Benchekroun et al., 2003). It is a potent and selective inhibitor of phosphodiesterase type 5 enzymes that acts to break down cyclic guanosine monophosphate (cGMP) (Boolell et al., 1996). The medication amplifies the effect of sexual stimulation by retarding the degradation of this enzyme. Sildenafil has been found effective in several subpopulations of men with erectile dysfunction, including sufferers from diabetes (Basu and Ryder, 2004), hypertension (Feldman et al., 1999), spinal cord injuries (Hultling et al., 2000; Deforge et al., 2006), multiple sclerosis (Fowler et al., 2005), depression (Seidman et al., 2001; Rosen et al., 2004; Tignol et al., 2004; Fava et al., 2006), PTSD (Orr et al., 2006), and schizophrenia (Aviv et al., 2004; Gopalakrishnan et al., 2006), men after resection of the prostate or radical prostatectomy (Nandipati et al., 2006), after renal transplant (Sharma et al., 2006), men on dialysis (Dachille et al., 2006), and men aged 65 years and older (Wagner et al., 2001; Carson, 2004).

Psychogenic erectile dysfunction (ED) patients are excellent candidates for sildenafil citrate therapy due to the intact neurovascular pathway. Nevertheless, the drug has been reported to be effective only in about 78% of patients with psychogenic ED (McMahon et al., 2000). It is likely that performance anxiety and sympathetic overtone are the cause of this unresponsiveness to sildenafil citrate during awakening, though data supporting this assumption are lacking (Rosen, 2001). The drug has been found to be effective and well tolerated in men with mild to moderate erectile dysfunction of no clinically identifiable organic cause (Eardley, 2001).

With the presence of PDE5 in choroidal and retinal vessels sildenafil citrate increase choroidal blood flow and cause vasodilation of the retinal vasculature. The most common symptoms are a blue tinge to vision and an increased sensitivity to light (Kerr and Danesh-Meyer, 2009). Adverse effects include headache, visual and retinal disturbances, dizziness and pupil-sparing third nerve palsy (Monastero et al., 2001). There have been reports of non-arteritic anterior ischaemic optic neuropathy and serous macular detachment in users of PDE5 inhibitors; although a causal relationship has not been conclusively shown. Despite the role of cGMP in the production and drainage of aqueous humor these medications do not appear to alter intraocular pressure and are safe in patients with glaucoma. All PDE5 inhibitors weakly inhibit PDE6 located in rod and cone photoreceptors resulting in mild and transient visual symptoms that correlate with plasma concentrations. Psychophysical tests reveal no effect on visual acuity, visual fields or contrast sensitivity; however, some studies show a mild and reversible impairment of blue-green colour discrimination. PDE5 inhibitors transiently alter retinal function on electroretinogram testing but do not appear to be retinotoxic. Despite the role of cyclic nucleotides in tear production there is no detrimental effect on tear film quality. Based on the available evidence PDE5 inhibitors have a good ocular safety profile (Kerr and Danesh-Meyer, 2009).

It has been reported that sildenafil citrate significantly improves nocturnal penile erections in sildenafil non-responding patients with psychogenic erectile dysfunction (Abdel-Naser et al., 2004). Several pharmacological and physiological properties of sildenafil have been described (Cheitlin et al., 1999; Aviv et al., 2004; Galie et al., 2005; Hoeper et al., 2006)

In Nigeria, most individuals often use sildenafil citrate indiscriminately for sexual arousal. There is a growing apprehension that it could be harmful or injurious to the body. Though sildenafil is currently being used to treat erectile dysfunction in patients with multiple sclerosis, Parkinson disease, multisystem atrophy, and spinal cord injury by improving their neurologically related erectile dysfunction, conversely, it has been implicated in a number of neurological problems, such as intracerebral hemorrhage, migraine, seizure, transient global amnesia, nonarteritic anterior ischemic optic neuropathy, macular degeneration, branch retinal artery occlusion, and ocular muscle palsies. Thus, preclinical and very limited clinical data suggest that sildenafil may have therapeutic potential in selected neurological disorders. However, numerous reports are available regarding neurological adverse events ascribed to the drug. Although sildenafil shows some promise as a therapeutic agent in selected neurological disorders, well-designed clinical trials are needed before the agent can be recommended for use in any neurological disorder (Farooq et al., 2008).

The liver is the largest glandular organ of the body, weighing between 1.4-1.6kg. It lies below the diaphragm in the thoracic region of the abdomen. It plays a major role in metabolism and has a number of functions in the body, including glycogen storage, plasma protein synthesis, production of bile; an alkaline compound which aids in digestion, and detoxification of most substances (Gartner and Hiatt, 2000).

The Kidney is a paired organ located in the posterior abdominal wall, whose functions include the removal of waste products from the blood and regulation of the amount of fluid and electrolytes balance in the body. As in humans, the majority of drugs administered are eliminated by a combination of hepatic metabolism and renal excretion (Katzung 1998). The kidney also plays a major role in drug metabolism, but its major importance to drugs is still its excretory functions.

Since the liver and kidneys are involved in the performance of these varied functions they may be susceptible to injury particularly in situation of toxicity. This work is carried out to investigate the histological effects of Sildenafil citrate on the liver and kidneys of adult Wistar rat. Though there are little or no literature report of toxicity of this drug on these two organs, but because they are vital organs in the body it is worthwhile to study its effects on them. Though Daghfous et al., in 2005 reported that sildenafil-induced liver disease.

This study will further corroborate or disprove the toxic effects of Sildenafil citrate in organs other than sex organs, with a view to advising the consumers on the inherent dangers of excessive consumption of the aphrodisiac.

2. Materials and methods

Twenty-four (24) adult Wistar rats of both sexes, weighing between 220.5g and 233.8g, with an average weight of 222.3g were randomly assigned into three treatment (n=18) and control (n=6) groups. The rats were obtained and maintained in the Animal holdings of the Department of Anatomy, School of Basic Medical Sciences, University of Benin, Benin city, Nigeria. They were fed with growers' mash obtained from Edo feed and flour mill limited, Ewu, Edo State and given water and feed ad libitum. The rats were acclimatized for 4 weeks before the experiment started.

2.1 Sildenafil citrate administration

The rats in the treatment groups (A, B, & C) received respectively, 0.25mg/kg, 0.70mg/kg and 1.43mg/kg body weight of Sildenafil citrate base dissolved in distilled water daily for 6 weeks, through orogastric feeding tube, while that of the control group D, received equal volume of distilled water daily during the period of the experiment. The rats were sacrificed by cervical dislocation on day forty-three of the experiment. The liver and kidneys of the animals in each group were dissected out and quickly fixed in 10% formal saline for general histological studies.

2.2 Histological study

The liver and Kidney tissues were dehydrated in an ascending grade of alcohol (ethanol), cleared in xylene and embedded in paraffin wax. Serial sections of 7 microns thick were obtained using a rotatory microtome. The deparaffinised sections were stained routinely with hematoxylin and eosin reagent. Photomicrographs of the specimens were obtained using digital research photographic microscope in the University of Benin research laboratory.

2.3 Liver enzyme assay and other metabolic panel

Blood samples were collected from all the rats within different treatment groups through the orbital venous plexuses on the last day of the experiment under chloroform anaesthesia. Blood serum was separated by centrifugation at 3000 rpm for 15 min. Serum was analysed colorimetrically for total protein, albumin, transaminases (aspartate aminotransferase (AST) and alanine aminotransferase (ALT). Blood samples were also collected and analyzed for blood urea nitrogen (BUN) and serum creatinine (Scr) by using the commercial kits (McClatchey, 1994)

2.4 Approval

This study was given consent and approval for the methodology and other ethical issues concerning the work by the University of Benin Research Ethics Ccommittee.

2.5 Statistical analysis

The results were expressed as mean ±SD. Data obtained from liver function test, blood urea nitrogen (BUN) and serum creatinine (Scr) were subjected to statistical analysis using one way analysis of variance (ANOVA) then followed with post hoc test (Least Square Deviation), P value of less than 0.05 was considered significant.

3. Results

3.1 Liver tissue

The control sections of the liver showed normal histological features with the hepatic lobules showing irregular hexagonal boundary defined by portal tract and sparse collagenous tissues. The hepatic portal veins, bile ductules and hepatic artery within the portal tract were all visible (Figure 1).

The treatment sections of the liver showed some histological changes that were at variance with those obtained in the control. There were evidence of dilatations of the central veins, which contained lysed red blood cells and cyto-architectural distortions of the hepatocytes and centrilobular haemorrhagic necrosis. There were atrophic and degenerative changes with the group that received 1.43mg/kg body weight of Sildenafil citrate more (Figure 2, 3 & 4).

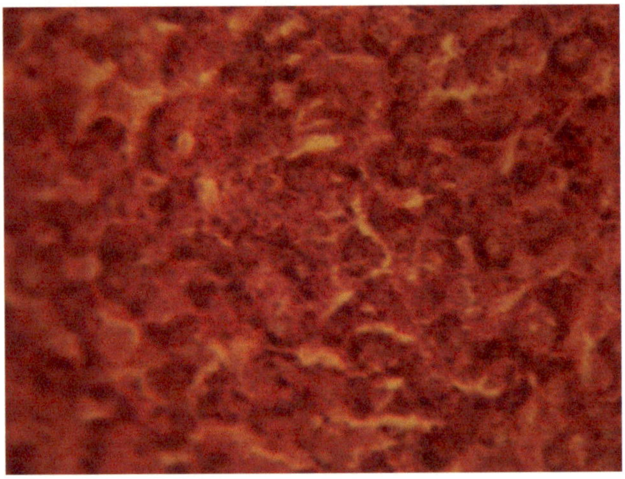

Fig. 1. Control section of the liver. Group 'D' (Mag. X400)

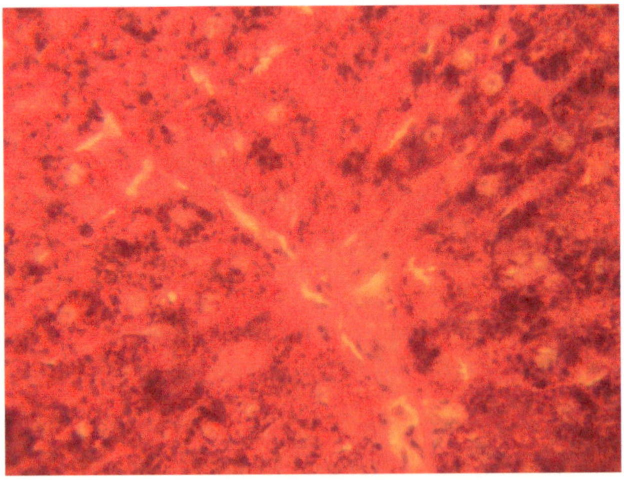

Fig. 2. Photomicrograph of the liver showing in the treatment groups 'A' that received 0.25mg/kg body weight of Sildenafil citrate. It shows portal tract and sparse collagenous tissues. The liver sinusoid and central veins were visible (Mag. x400)

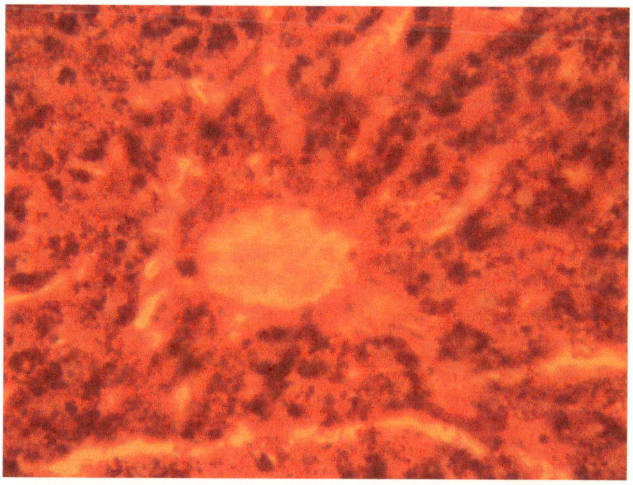

Fig. 3. Photomicrograph of the liver showing in the treatment groups 'B' that received 0.70mg/kg body weight of Sildenafil citrate. There were atrophic and degenerative changes around the hepatocytes and central vein, which was dilated and contained lysed red blood cell (Mag. X400).

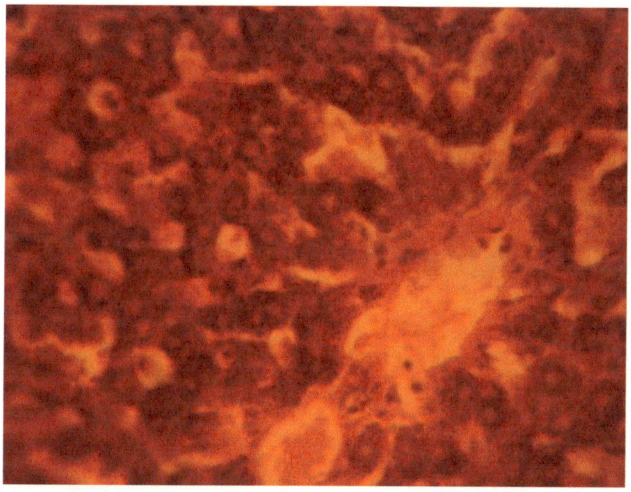

Fig. 4. Photomicrograph of the liver showing in the treatment groups 'C' that received 1.43mg/kg body weight of Sildenafil citrate. There were marked atrophic and degenerative changes around the hepatocytes and lysed red blood cell containing dilated central vein (Mag. X400).

3.2 Kidney tissue

The control sections of the kidneys showed normal histological features. The section indicated a detailed cortical parenchyma and the renal corpuscles appeared as dense rounded structures with the glomerulus surrounded by a narrow Bowman's spaces (Figure 5)

The kidneys of the animals in group 'A' treated with 0.25mg/kg of Sildenafil citrate revealed some level of cyto-architectural distortion of the cortical structures as compared to the control (Figure 6)

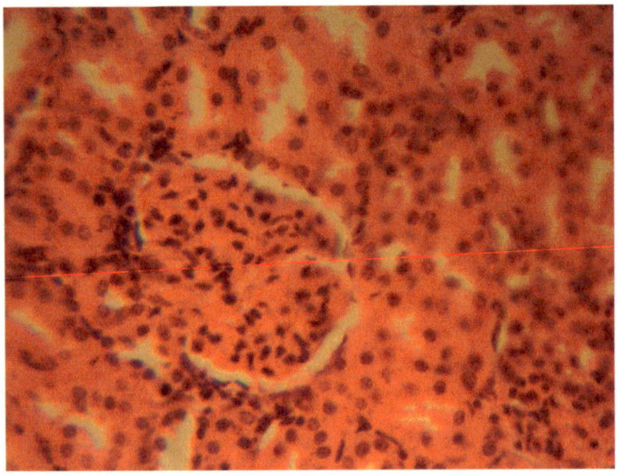

Fig. 5. Control section of the Kidney. Group 'D' (Mag. X400)

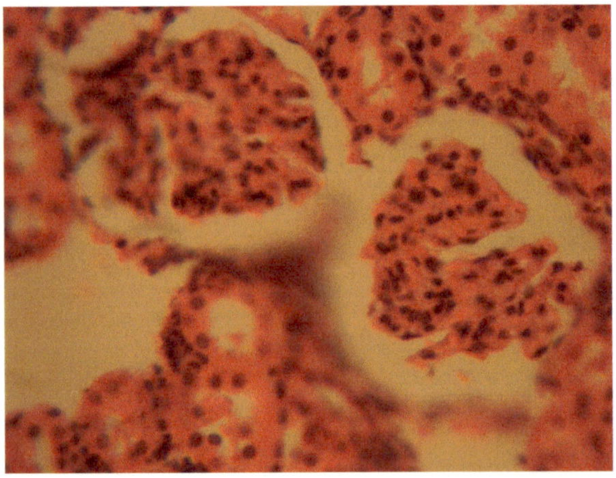

Fig. 6. Photomicrograph of the Kidney showing in the treatment groups 'A' that received 0.25mg/kg body weight of Sildenafil citrate showing some level of cyto-architectural distortion of the cortical structures (Mag. X400)

The kidney sections of animals in group 'B' treated with 0.70mg/kg of Sildenafil citrate revealed mild to moderate distortion of cyto-architecture of the renal cortical structures with mild degenerative and atrophic changes. The kidney sections of animals in group 'C' treated with 1.43mg/kg of Sildenafil citrate revealed marked distortion of cyto-architecture of the renal cortical structures, and degenerative and atrophic changes. There were vacuolations appearing in the stroma and loss of renal corpuscles which were less identified and the Bowman's spaces were sparsely distributed as compared to the control group 'D' (Figure 7)

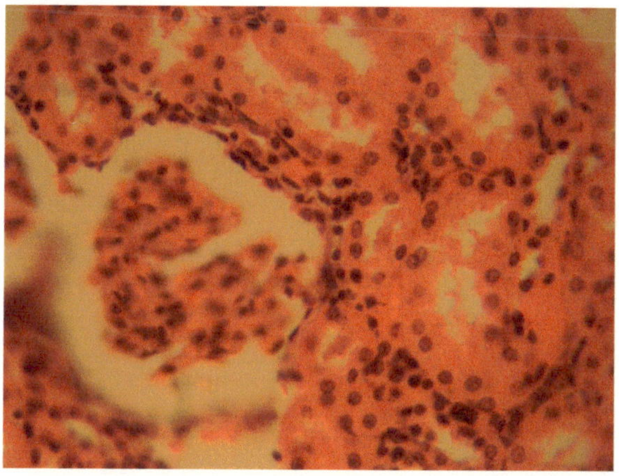

Fig. 7. Photomicrograph of the Kidney showing in the treatment groups 'B' that received 0.70mg/kg body weight of Sildenafil citrate mild to moderate distortion of cyto-architecture of the renal cortical structures with mild degenerative and atrophic changes (Mag. X400)

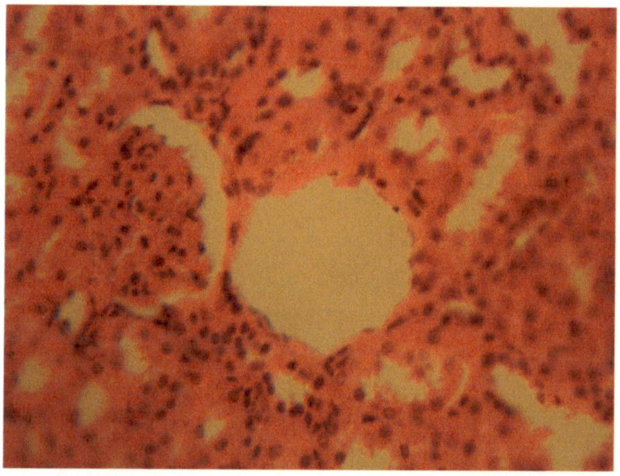

Fig. 8. Photomicrograph of the Kidney showing in the treatment groups 'B' that received 1.43mg/kg body weight of Sildenafil citrate marked distortion of cyto-architecture of the renal cortical structures, and degenerative and atrophic changes. There were vacuolations appearing in the stroma and loss of renal corpuscles which were less identified and the Bowman's spaces were sparsely distributed.

Table 1 below shows the mean and standard deviation of each group for the different components. The table revealed that experimental group C (Exp. C) has the highest mean for components: Total Protein, Albumin, ALT and AST. The Control group had the least mean for all the components.

Table 2 shows the analysis of variance for the four groups for the five components. The results revealed that the difference between the means of the four groups for each component is significant ($P < 0.0001$).

The result of this experiment revealed that Sildenafil citrate consumption caused significant ($P<0.05$) increase in functional nephrotoxicity indicators such as BUN and Serum creatinin in Sildenafil citrate-treated rats compared with control (Table 3).

	Group	N	Mean	Std. Deviation	Std. Error
Protein (g/dl)	Control	6	4.46	0.59	0.19
	Exp. A	6	5.73	0.21	0.04
	Exp. B	6	6.69	0.37	0.10
	Exp. C	6	7.73	0.42	0.12
	Total	24	6.68	0.98	0.22
Albumin (g/dl)	Control	6	2.83	0.38	0.16
	Exp. A	6	3.45	0.26	0.07
	Exp. B	6	4.31	0.29	0.09
	Exp. C	6	5.23	0.34	0.13
	Total	24	3.66	0.69	0.17
ALT (µmol/l)	Control	6	32.42	0.51	0.26
	Exp. A	6	73.84	11.63	4.34
	Exp. B	6	108.66	27.03	8.60
	Exp. C	6	112.73	29.42	9.71
	Total	24	78.34	35.20	7.84
AST (µmol/l)	Control	6	13.60	0.61	0.28
	Exp. A	6	58.70	8.84	3.16
	Exp. B	6	79.82	29.37	9.90
	Exp. C	6	88.57	32.62	11.72
	Total	24	53.16	35.45	6.84

Table 1. Descriptive statistics, protein and some liver enzymes assay of groups.

	Source of Variation	Sum of Squares	df	Mean Square	F	Sig.
Protein	Between Groups	17.612	3	8.560	91.528	.000
	Within groups	1.978	21	0.096		
	Total	18.282	24			
Albumin	Between Groups	7.749	3	3.471	60.21	.000
	Within groups	1.881	21	0.083		
	Total	8.976	24			
ALT	Between Groups	19421.463	3	9823.571	31.791	.000
	Within groups	5627.238	21	302.135		
	Total	25570.766	24			
AST	Between Groups	13873.376	3	6936.688	23.022	.000
	Within groups	5724.897	21	301.310		
	Total	18.898	24			

P <0.0001

Table 2. Analysis of Variance (ANOVA) of the Four Groups

	BUN (mg/dl)	Scr (mg/dl)
Control	14.38±2.5	0.47±0.21
Experimental group A (0.25mg/kg)	28.7±4.63	2.3±0.23
Experimental group B (0.70mg/kg)	55±0.72	3.2±0.99
Experimental group C (1.43mg/kg)	69±0.33	3.8±2.62

Table 3. Effects of Sildenafil citrate consumption on BUN and Scr concentration

4. Discussion

The results of the histological studies revealed that with increasing dose of Sildenafil citrate consumption, there were varying degrees of dilatations of the central vein of the liver which contained lysed red blood cells in the treatment group compared to the control sections of the liver, and as well as varying degree of cyto-architectural distortion and reduction in the number of renal corpuscle in the kidneys of the treated groups compared to the control sections of the kidneys. This suggests that the distortion of the cyto-architecture of the liver could be associated with functional changes that may be detrimental to the health of the rats. The proliferating cells of the liver, which produce red and white blood cells, are normally found between the hepatic cells and the walls of the vessels (Singh, 1997).

As a result of the distortion and dilatation of the hepatocytes and their central vein, the haematopoietic function of the liver may have been highly affected as a result of probable toxic effect of Sildenafil citrate. This was further buttressed by the increase in the liver enzymes obtained in the test group. In addition, total protein and albumin increased in this study the increase in total protein may be due to the fact that Sildenafil citrate was given for a short period of time. The resultant effect is acute toxicity leading to enhanced hepato-cellullar activity and increase in globulin and albumin components of the protein .However, with prolonged usage, hepatic necrosis is likely to occur with a resultant low albumin levels.

There were several diffuse degeneration and necrosis of the tubular epithelial cells in the kidneys of the treated animals. The degenerative and atrophic changes where observed more in the kidneys of rats that received the highest dose (1.43mg/kg) of Sildenafil citrate.

It may be inferred from the present results that higher doses of Sildenafil citrate consumption may have resulted in degenerative and atrophic changes observed in the renal corpuscle. The possible deduction from these results is that secondary metabolites, which are largely responsible for therapeutic or pharmacological activities of medicinal plants (Perry, 1980), may also account for their toxicity when the dosage is abused.

Pathological or accidental cell death is regarded as necrotic and could result from extrinsic insults to the cell as osmotic thermal, toxic and traumatic effect (Farber et al, 1981). Physiological cell death is regarded as apoptotic and organized programmed cell death (PCD) that is mediated by active and intrinsic mechanisms. The process of cellular necrosis involves disruption of membranes, as well as structural and functional integrity. Cellular necrosis is not induced by stimuli intrinsic to the cells as in programmed cell death (PCD), but by an abrupt environmental perturbation and departure from the normal physiological conditions (Farber et al, 1981).

Cellular degeneration has been reported to result in cell death, which is of two types, namely apoptotic and necrotic cell death. These two types differ morphologically and biochemically (Wyllie, 1980). Pathological or accidental cell death is regarded as necrotic and could result from extrinsic insults to the cell such as osmotic, thermal, toxic and traumatic effects (Wyllie, 1980). Cell death in response to toxins occurs as a controlled event involving a genetic programme in which caspase enzymes are activated (Waters et al., 1994).

As the hepatocytes swell as seen in this study the activities of cellular transporters are approximately modified by up or down regulations as earlier reported in the case of hyponatraemia or hypernatraemia (Johnson, 1995). Ischaemic or pharmacologic disruption of cellular transporters can cause swelling of parenchyma of the liver cells. Sildenafil citrate may have acted as toxins to the hepatocytes, thereby affecting their cellular integrity and causing defect in membrane permeability and cell volume homeostasis.

The actual mechanism by which Sildenafil citrate induced cellular degeneration observed in this experiment needs further investigation. The necrosis observed is probably due to the high concentration of Sildenafil citrate on the liver and kidney; this obviously will affect the normal detoxification, excretory processes and other functions of the liver and kidneys respectively.

The limitation of this study was the duration of study (acute) as opposed to chronic which could have yielded more light on the pathology.

5. Conclusion

The results obtained in this study following the administration of 0.25mg/kg, 0.70mg/kg and 1.43mg/kg per day of Sildenafil to adult Wistar rats affected the histology of the liver and kidneys. These results suggest that the functions of the liver and kidney may have been adversely affected. It is recommended that caution should therefore be advocated in the intake of this product and further studies be carried out to examine these findings.

6. References

[1] Abdel-Naser MB, Imam A, Wollina U (2004). Sildenafil citrate significantly improves nocturnal penile erections in sildenafil non-responding patients with psychogenic erectile dysfunction. Int. J. Impot. Res. 16, 552–556.

[2] Aviv A, Shelef A, Weizman A (2004). An open-label trial of sildenafil addition in risperidone-treated male schizophrenia patients with erectile dysfunction. Journal of Clinical Psychiatry 65:97–103.

[3] Basu A, Ryder RE (2004). New treatment options for erectile dysfunction in patients with diabetes mellitus. Drugs, 64:2667–2688.

[4] Benchekroun A, Faik M, Benjelloun S (2003). A baseline-controlled, open-label, flexible dose-escalation study to assess the safety and efficacy of sildenafil citrate (Viagra) in patients with erectile dysfunction. Int. J Impot. Res. 15(Suppl. 1):S19–S24

[5] Boolell M, Allen MJ, Ballard SA (1996). Oral sildenafil: an orally active type 5 cyclic GMP specific phosphodiesterase inhibitor for the treatment of penile erectile dysfunction. Int J Impot Res; 8: 47–52.

[6] Carson CC (2004). Erectile dysfunction: evaluation and new treatment options. Psychosomatic Medicine, 66:664–671.

[7] Cheitlin MD, Hutter AM, Brindis RG, Kaul S, Russell RO, Zusman RM (1999). Use of sildenafil (Viagra) in patients with cardiovascular disease. *Circulation*, 99:168–177.

[8] Cunningham AV, Smith KH (2001). Anterior ischemic optic neuropathy associated with Viagra. *Journal of Neuro-Ophthalmology, 21*, 22–25.

[9] Dachille G, Pagliarulo V, Ludovico GM (2006). Sexual dysfunction in patients under dialytic treatment. Minerva Urologica e Nefrologica 58:195–200.

[10] Deforge D, Blackmer J, Garritty C (2006). Male erectile dysfunction following spinal cord injury: a systematic review. *Spinal Cord*, 44:465–473.
[11] Drury RAB, Wallington EA, Cameron R. Carleton's Histological Techniques: 4th ed., Oxford University Press NY. U.S.A. 1967 279-280.
[12] Eardley I (2001). Efficacy and safety of sildenafil citrate in the treatment of men with mild to moderate erectile dysfunction The British Journal of Psychiatry. 178: 325-330
[13] Farber JL Chein KR, Mittnacht S (1981). The pathogenesis of Irreversible cell injury in ischemia. American Journal of Pathology; 102:271-281.
[14] Farooq MU, Naravetla B, Moore PW, Majid A, Gupta R, Kassab MY (2008). Role of Sildenafil in Neurological Disorders Clinical Neuropharmacology: Vol 31 - Issue 6 - pp 353-362
[15] Fava M, Nurnberg HG, Seidman SN (2006). Efficacy and safety of sildenafil in men with serotonergic antidepressant-associated erectile dysfunction: results from a randomized, double-blind, placebo-controlled trial. J. Clin Psych., 67:240–246.
[16] Feldman R, Meuleman EJ, Steers W (1999). Sildenafil citrate (VIAGRA) in the treatment of erectile dysfunction: analysis of two flexible dose-escalation studies. Sildenafil Study Group. Int. J Clin Pract, 53(Suppl. 102):10–12.
[17] Fowler CJ, Miller JR, Sharief MK (2005). A double blind, randomised study of sildenafil citrate for erectile dysfunction in men with multiple sclerosis. J Neuro. Neurosurg Psych., 76:700–705.
[18] Galie N, Ghofrani HA, Torbicki A, Barst RJ, Rubin LJ, Badesch D, Fleming T, Parpia T, Burgess G, Branzi A, Grimminger F, Kurzyna M, Simonneau G (2005). Sildenafil citrate therapy for pulmonary arterial hypertension. *N Engl J Med* Nov 17; 353:2148-57.
[19] Gartner LP, Hiatt JL (2000). Color Atlas of Histology; 3rd Edi., Lippincott Williams & Wilkins Publishers, A Wolters Kluwer company, pp 294-301.
[20] Goldstein I, Lue TF, Padma-Nathan H, Rosen RC, Steers WD, Wicker PA (1998). Oral sildenafil in the treatment of erectile dysfunction. N Engl J Med; 338: 1397–1404.
[21] Gopalakrishnan R, Jacob KS, Kuruvilla A (2006). Sildenafil in the treatment of antipsychotic-induced erectile dysfunction: a randomized, double-blind, placebo-controlled, flexible-dose, two-way crossover trial. American Journal of Psychiatry, 163:494–499.
[22] Hoeper MM, Welte T, Izbicki G, Rosengarten D, Picard E, Kuschner WG, Galiè N, Rubin LJ, Simonneau G (2006). Sildenafil Citrate Therapy for Pulmonary Arterial Hypertension. N Engl J Med; 354:1091-1093.
[23] Hultling C, Giuliano F, Quirk F (2000). Quality of life in patients with spinal cord injury receiving Viagra (sildenafil citrate) for the treatment of erectile dysfunction. Spinal Cord, 38:363–370.
[24] Johnson CE (1995). Effects of fluid imbalances In: Neurosciences in Medicine. Conn MP (Ed).New York: JB Lippincott Company; 187-189.
[25] Katzung BG (1998). Basic and Clinical Pharmacology 7th edition, Appleton and Lange, Stamford CT; pp. 372-375
[26] Kerr NM, Danesh-Meyer HV (2009). Phosphodiesterase inhibitors and the eye. Clinical & Experimental Ophthalmology, Volume 37 Issue 5, Pages 514 - 523
[27] Daghfous R, El Aidli S, Zaiem A, Loueslati MH, Belkahia C (2005). Sildenafil-Associated Hepatotoxicity. The American Journal of Gastroenterology 100, 1895–1896; doi:10.1111/j.1572- 0241.41983_6.x
[28] Martins LJ, Al-Abdulla NA, Kirsh JR, Sieber FE, Portera-Cailliau C (1998). Neurodegeneration in excitotoxicity, global cerebral ischemia and target

deprivation: A perspective on the contributions of apoptosis and necrosis. Brain Res. Bull. 46(4): 281-309.
[29] McClatchey KD (1994). Clinical Laboratory Medicine London Williams & Wilkins;
[30] McMahon CG, Samali R, Johnson H (2000). Efficacy, safety and patient acceptance of sildenafil citrate as treatment for erectile dysfunction. J Urol; 164: 1192–1196.
[31] Monatero R, Pipia C, Camarda LKC, Camarda R (2001). Intracerebral haemorrhage associated with sildenafil citrate, J. Neurol., Vol. 248: 2; 141-142.
[32] Nandipati KC, Raina R, Agarwal A, Zippe CD (2006). Erectile dysfunction following radical retropubic prostatectomy: epidemiology, pathophysiology and pharmacological management. Drugs & Aging, 23:101–117.
[33] Orr G, Weiser M, Polliack M (2006). Effectiveness of sildenafil in treating erectile dysfunction in PTSD patients: a double-blind, placebo-controlled crossover study. Journal of Clinical Psychopharmacology, 26:426–430.
[34] Perry LM (1980). Medicinal plants of East and South East Asia, MIT Press, Cambridge Massachusetts.
[35] Pomeranz HD, Smith KH, Hart WM, Jr, Egan RA (2002). Sildenafil-associated nonarteric anterior ischemic optic neuropathy. *Ophthalmology, 109,* 584–587.
[36] Pomeranz HD, Bhavsar AR (2005). Nonarteric ischemic optic neuropathy developing soon after use of sildenafil (Viagra): A report of seven new cases. *Journal of Neuro-Ophthalmology, 25,* 9–13.
[37] Rosen RC (2001). Psychogenic erectile dysfunction. Classification and management. Urol Clin North Am; 28: 269–278.
[38] Rosen RC, Seidman SN, Menza MA (2004). Quality of life, mood, and sexual function: a path analytic model of treatment effects in men with erectile dysfunction and depressive symptoms. Int J Impot Res, 16:334–340.
[39] Seidman SN, Roose SP, Menza MA (2001). Treatment of erectile dysfunction in men with depressive symptoms: results of a placebo-controlled trial with sildenafil citrate. American Journal of Psychiatry, 158:1623–1630.
[40] Sharma RK, Prasad N, Gupta A, Kapoor R (2006). Treatment of erectile dysfunction with sildenafil citrate in renal allograft recipients: a randomized, double-blind, placebo-controlled, crossover trial. American Journal of Kidney Diseases, 48:128–133.
[41] Siesjo BK (1978). Utilization of substrates by brain tissues, (In) Brain energy metabolism. John Wiley & Sons, USA. 101-130.
[42] Singh I (1997). Textbook of Human Histology with color atlas 3rd edn. New Delhi: Jaypee Brothers Medical Publishers Ltd; 238-244.
[43] Tignol J, Furlan PM, Gomez-Beneyto M (2004). Efficacy of sildenafil citrate (Viagra) for the treatment of erectile dysfunction in men in remission from depression. International Clinical Psychopharmacology, 19:191–199.
[44] Wagner G, Montorsi F, Auerbach S, Collins M (2001). Sildenafil citrate (VIAGRA) improves erectile function in elderly patients with erectile dysfunction: a subgroup analysis. Journal of Gerontology: Biological Sciences and Medical Sciences, 56:M113–M119.
[45] Waters CM, Wakinshaw G, Moser B, Mitchell IJ (1994). Death of neurons in the neonatal rodent globus pallidus occurs as a mechanism of apoptosis. Neuroscience: 63: 881-894.
[46] Wyllie AH (1980). Glucocorticoid-induced thymocyte apoptosis is associated with endogenous endonuclease activation. Nature: 284:555- 556.